Developing
Reflective Practice

A Guide for Students and Practitioners
of Health and Social Care

Health and Social Care titles available from Lantern Publishing Ltd

Clinical Skills for Student Nurses edited by Robin Richardson
ISBN 978 1 906052 04 1
Understanding Research and Evidence-based Practice by Bruce Lindsay
ISBN 978 1 906052 01 0
Values for Care Practice by Sue Cuthbert and Jan Quallington
ISBN 978 1 906052 05 8
Communication and Interpersonal Skills by Elaine Donnelly and Lindsey Neville
ISBN 978 1 906052 06 5
Numeracy, Clinical Calculations and Basic Statistics by Neil Davison
ISBN 978 1 906052 07 2
Essential Study Skills edited by Marjorie Lloyd and Peggy Murphy
ISBN 978 1 906052 14 0
Safe and Clean Care by Tina Tilmouth with Simon Tilmouth
ISBN 978 1 906052 08 9
Neonatal Care edited by Amanda Williamson and Kenda Crozier
ISBN 978 1 906052 09 6
Fundamentals of Diagnostic Imaging edited by Anne-Marie Dixon
ISBN 978 1 906052 10 2
Fundamentals of Nursing Care by Anne Llewellyn and Sally Hayes
ISBN 978 1 906052 13 3
The Care and Wellbeing of Older People edited by Angela Kydd, Tim Duffy and
    F.J. Raymond Duffy
ISBN 978 1 906052 15 7
Palliative Care edited by Elaine Stevens and Janette Edwards
ISBN 978 1 906052 16 4
Nursing in the UK: A Handbook for Nurses from Overseas by Wendy Benbow and
    Gill Jordan
ISBN 978 1 906052 00 3
Interpersonal Skills for the People Professions edited by Lindsey Neville
ISBN 978 1 906052 18 8
Understanding and Helping People in Crisis by Elaine Donnelly, Briony Williams and
    Tess Parkinson
ISBN 978 1 906052 21 8
A Handbook for Student Nurses by Wendy Benbow and Gill Jordan
ISBN 978 1 906052 19 5
Professional Practice in Public Health edited by Jill Stewart and Yvonne Cornish
ISBN 978 1 906052 20 1
Understanding Wellbeing edited by Anneyce Knight and Allan McNaught
ISBN 978 1 908625 00 7

Developing
Reflective Practice

A Guide for Students and Practitioners of Health and Social Care

Natius Oelofsen

Lantern

ISBN: 978 1 908625 01 4

First published in 2012 by Lantern Publishing Limited

Lantern Publishing Limited, The Old Hayloft, Vantage Business Park, Bloxham Road, Banbury OX16 9UX, UK

www.lanternpublishing.com

British Library Cataloguing in Publication Data
A catalogue record for this book is available from the British Library

The authors and publisher have made every attempt to ensure the content of this book is up to date and accurate. However, healthcare knowledge and information is changing all the time so the reader is advised to double-check any information in this text on drug usage, treatment procedures, the use of equipment, etc. to confirm that it complies with the latest safety recommendations, standards of practice and legislation, as well as local Trust policies and procedures. Students are advised to check with their tutor and/or mentor before carrying out any of the procedures in this textbook.

Typeset by Phoenix Photosetting, Chatham, UK
Cover design by Andrew Magee Design Ltd
Printed and bound by MPG Books Ltd, Bodmin, UK
Distributed by NBN International, 10 Thornbury Road, Plymouth, PL6 7PP, UK

This book is dedicated to two very special people in my life:

My father, Willem Oelofsen (1936–2011) who taught me so much about life and what is really important; and Eucharia, my wife, who is my constant inspiration.

CONTENTS

PREFACE

The idea for this book emerged from a series of structured, topic-based reflective practice sessions that I was invited to facilitate in various organisations over the last four years. The monthly groups were run for staff who worked in settings as diverse as a children's home, a nursery, Sure Start children's centres, and a team who provided intensive input to multi-problem families. Although the settings were diverse and participants had a wide range of qualifications, the groups all responded well to a very consistent set of session topics. This alerted me to the need of practitioners who work with vulnerable people in a range of settings to develop a conceptual understanding of the psychological processes which they are likely to encounter during the course of their work. Feedback from participants informed the choice of topics that were covered in these groups and this is also reflected in the chapter topics of this book.

Group sessions were also designed to enable participants to reflect on the impact of the issues at hand or the session topic on themselves and their own practice. Exercises were designed to foster experiential learning and group problem solving with the ultimate aim of improving practice. This approach was also followed when reflective activities were developed for this book.

Developing reflective practice in frontline settings involves several key players. First of all there are individual practitioners who need to be open to learn new concepts and ideas, reflect how these apply to themselves and their practice, and how they can improve the quality of their own work as a result. Managers within services are important as they are the catalysts for developing reflective teams. In particular, their openness to questions about accepted ways of doing things is a crucial factor in determining whether or not reflection can lead to positive change. Finally, organisations are only able to benefit from reflective practitioners and reflective teams once pathways for constructive feedback are created and allowed to influence organisational culture and practice. In the original reflective practice groups referred to above, the groups and I spent much time reflecting on how their insights into their own practices could be used within supervision and through other routes to influence and foster team and organisation-based change. Many of the following chapters include reflective activities that were designed to help practitioners reflect on organisational factors that influence their practice and also consider ways in which to influence practice for the better.

This book was written in the hope that making the material that others found helpful more widely available may enable large numbers of practitioners in frontline settings to become more reflective. But the ultimate aim of reflective practice is always to improve practice, and therefore it is my sincere hope that this book will become a useful tool to help frontline services improve the quality of what they offer to those who are vulnerable in our society.

Natius Oelofsen

December 2011

ABOUT THE AUTHOR

Dr Natius Oelofsen is a consultant clinical psychologist trained in South Africa and the UK. He has worked in the UK's National Health Service as a clinical psychologist since 1998 in a variety of settings, including child and adolescent mental health, child development/paediatrics, and he is currently a consultant in an adult learning disability service.

In addition to his clinical practice, Natius also works as a psychologist, trainer and consultant to a variety of public and third-sector organisations that provide services to children and families, including practitioners in children's centres, nurseries, children's homes and respite provision for disabled children. He has run reflective practice groups and team-based training for senior practitioners and managers in a range of health and social care providers.

Further details of the training in reflective practice that Natius offers can be seen at www.reflective-learning.co.uk.

ACKNOWLEDGEMENTS

No project of this magnitude can come to fruition without the efforts of a large number of people. Although space does not permit me to thank everyone, I would like to acknowledge the contributions of the following:

First of all, I owe a debt of gratitude to all the members of the reflective practice groups I was fortunate enough to facilitate over the past four years. Your enthusiastic participation and eagerness to engage with new ideas were the reasons for writing this book.

Secondly, I would like to thank all the commissioning managers in the various organisations that commissioned reflective practice groups for their staff. I am so grateful that you believed in what I had to offer your teams. In particular, I would like to mention the following: Lorraine Cartwright, Sheri Wilks, Suzie Turner-Jones, Julie Hartnell and Alison Gillies for your belief in the concept and your support over the years.

I gratefully acknowledge the assistance provided by Belbin Associates in compiling the Team Roles section of Chapter 11 and for permission to use descriptions of the Belbin Team Roles®. Jessica Kingsley Publishers kindly gave permission to use copyrighted material from one of their publications in Chapter 12. A note of thanks also to Rebecca Button, Trainee Psychologist, who alerted me to a number of useful references relevant to the material covered in Chapter 5.

The process that lead from the inception to the completion of this project involved a number of individuals whose advice and support were invaluable: Judith Harvey from Reflect Press initially took on the project and got things off the ground, while Peter Oates and the team at Lantern Publishing saw the book through its final edits and the production stage. They are responsible for the beautifully produced book you now hold in your hands. Several anonymous reviewers provided thoughtful and, at times, challenging comments, while always upholding the inherent value of the book. Your suggestions contributed much to the end result. Many thanks.

I would also like to thank my family for their support. I am grateful to my wife, Eucharia, for believing in this book long before it was written and her encouragement throughout the process of writing. Many an hour of family time went into this project. Thank you for so graciously letting me write. To my young son, Nico: you demonstrate on a daily basis the curiosity and eagerness to learn that epitomises the best reflective practice. My parents also deserve a very special mention. Their interest in the progress of this project was a constant source of support. I am only sad that my father passed away before he could see the end result.

Finally, I was incredibly fortunate to be able to draw on so many great ideas from such a variety of sources throughout the chapters that follow. To all of these sources my sincere thanks. Any errors, omissions, or misperceptions are, of course, my own.

INTRODUCTION

This book was written as a companion for practitioners and students in health and social care on their journeys to becoming reflective practitioners. Reflective practice encompasses a variety of practices designed to help people make sense of their experiences in professional contexts. The material in this book is suitable for students and practitioners in a variety of fields, including nursing, psychology, social work, therapeutic child care, and education. What all of these fields have in common is that practitioners deal with fundamental human needs such as physical and mental health, housing, and education. Students on placement as well as qualified and experienced practitioners can benefit from reading this book and working through the reflective exercises that accompany the text.

The perspective taken here is very specifically a psychological one. Helping practitioners feel confident and competent involves both personal growth and a process of learning that enhances their confidence when confronted with complex and emotionally demanding situations in the workplace. While most training courses endeavour to prepare students to enter professional practice with a relevant skill set, it has been my observation that practitioners on the front line need to have access to a set of broader perspectives than their profession-specific theories and models to draw on when situations become complex. For reflective practice to be a truly empowering activity that improves the quality and sophistication of practice, while at the same time improving the confidence of practitioners, it should equip frontline staff with the ability to make sense of complexity and generate ideas for action that follow logically from an enhanced understanding of the situations on which they have reflected. This involves developing a sophisticated understanding of the interplay between individual, systemic, and organisational factors, as well as developing a strong sense of the impact of their own dynamics on these processes. This book therefore focuses on enhancing practitioners' understanding of the psychological dynamics involved in case work in frontline practice.

Another cornerstone of the philosophy underpinning this book is that becoming a reflective practitioner involves a process of personal growth. Reflective practitioners understand the assumptions inherent in their own approaches to practice. They are able to articulate and work with their own assumptions and attributions regarding their experiences in the workplace. This book contains structured exercises for reflection that aim to enhance such personal growth.

WHAT YOU CAN EXPECT FROM READING THIS BOOK

You should gain a thorough understanding of what reflective practice is and how it can benefit you and your team in their work. You can expect to become skilled at a variety of practical reflective methods and familiar with a range of ideas and approaches that will enable you to understand the psychological forces at play in your work. Your reflective journey is also likely to lead to a greater self-understanding as there are opportunities for you to learn more about your own functioning throughout the various chapters.

Apart from learning about different approaches, you can also expect to gain some practice at conceptualising your work with vulnerable people. You may develop a useful new vocabulary that has been designed to enable you to articulate your own and others' reactions to situations you encounter in the course of delivering services in ways that foster professional understanding and positive change. You can expect to work in new ways with your clients, helping them to become more reflective themselves and more open to new possibilities and positive change.

You will learn about stress management, preventing burnout, and how to make good use of supervision. Following your journey through this book, you should also have an enhanced awareness of yourself as a change agent and be able to use your personal reactions to service users to effect positive change.

HOW TO GET THE MOST OUT OF THIS BOOK

This book is designed to be suitable for both individuals and groups to work through. One of the key features of each chapter is a journal exercise chosen to facilitate individual reflection. Most of the other learning activities and exercises can be done individually, as part of a reflective group, or within your own team. One of the assumptions in this book is that people learn to reflect more effectively if they create opportunities to reflect in interaction with their peers. However, not everyone has ready access to a suitable group of peers, and therefore this book has been designed to offer opportunities for both individual and group reflection.

If you are a student working through this book, here are a few tips that might help you make the most of your experience:

- Try to apply the material in the different chapters to practical situations such as when you are on placement.

- Sometimes the most profound learning takes place when you start unpacking mundane experiences – examples include mapping out service users' journeys through a service, or focusing on someone's experience of first encountering a service.

- As a student you may have more opportunity than qualified practitioners to get a formal or informal group together to work through different chapters in this book. You should ask your placement supervisor if time can be made available while you are on placement for you to write a reflective journal (see *Chapter 2*).

- Finally, try to tackle at least some of the material every week. Working through the different chapters using a 'little and often' approach will benefit you more than trying to read whole chapters or even several chapters in one sitting.

STRUCTURE OF THIS BOOK

This book is divided into four parts. Part one introduces you to the concept of reflective practice and tells you how to reflect in practice. It explores what reflective practice is and introduces the three-stage reflective cycle that will be used in the rest of the book to structure the reflective process. It provides a practical toolkit of reflective methods, with worked examples that illustrate the methods discussed in the text.

Part two of the book aims to develop readers' understanding of the work they do within frontline settings by focusing on a selection of perspectives from psychology and psychotherapy. The topics covered were selected based on the kinds of issues I came across when facilitating reflective practice sessions in a range of health and social care settings. These settings included children's care services, family support practitioners based in children's centres, staff in a team working with complex multi-problem families, and staff in early years education. Topics covered include narrative approaches, attachment theory, the influence of cross-generational family history and migration, boundaries, facilitating change, and working ethically.

Part three reflects on the very important part that emotion plays within professional practice on the front line. People are emotional beings and practitioners in frontline services often experience strong emotions related to their work. So do users of services. The dynamics of the emotions that are aroused in practitioners and service users by each other and the various agencies involved with service users can have a profound impact on the way services are perceived and delivered. Perspectives on these issues are offered, primarily from the psychodynamic tradition.

The final part of the book deals with supporting frontline practice. Practitioners who themselves feel well-supported in their roles are likely to be more effective at providing the kinds of support expected of them by the users of their services. The topics in this section are effective team work, getting the most out of supervision, and dealing with stress and burnout.

Throughout each chapter there are practical exercises that readers can attempt alone or together with others. These exercises typically invite you to apply the material in the text to your setting. Throughout the text, different techniques and methods are introduced that might help you to reflect effectively on your practice. There are also four extended examples distributed throughout the book. These are worked examples, based on fictional scenarios that illustrate the concepts and techniques from the relevant chapters in the text.

TERMINOLOGY AND CASE EXAMPLES

The terms 'frontline services' and 'frontline organisations' are used to refer to all of those statutory, private, or voluntary sector services that support vulnerable people with their health, wellbeing, or social care needs.

The term 'service user' is used as a synonym for client, patient, customer, and any of the other terms that are currently in use to refer to people who access help from organisations in the community.

All case examples are fictional, although many have been adapted from actual situations. Names, identifying details, and settings have been changed to protect confidentiality.

HOW TO USE THIS BOOK

In each chapter, you will find a number of features that are included to make the book easier to use.

Chapter aims

These state the main learning outcomes you can expect from working through each chapter. Generally chapter aims follow the order of the headings in the chapter concerned and can therefore serve as a useful cue to guide you through the material in each chapter.

Reflective activities

These are the exercises for you to try. Some reflective activities can best be done on an individual basis, and some are more effective learning tools when used in a group setting. However, all of the reflective activities in this book can be adapted by readers for individual learning. To this end, I recommend that you start a reflective journal (see the section entitled *For the journal*, below).

Chapter summary

At the end of each chapter, I present a small number of key points (usually five) which are the core ideas I would like readers to take away from that chapter. These are intended to help you gain an overview of the relevant chapter and to identify material that you might wish to work through again.

For the journal

Each chapter contains an exercise for structured reflection. The topics of these exercises link directly to the material in the chapter, but might ask specific questions about how the issues raised in the chapter affect you in your individual setting. Some journal activities also challenge readers to involve their teams in small projects to improve services.

Further reading

These sections point readers to additional material that might be of interest, linked to the topic of each chapter. Where the full bibliographic reference to a recommended source is not given, the full reference can be found in the reference list.

PART ONE

INTRODUCING REFLECTIVE PRACTICE

01

REFLECTING ON REFLECTION: THEORIES AND PERSPECTIVES ON REFLECTIVE PRACTICE

THIS CHAPTER AIMS TO:

- Offer a definition of reflective practice and explain the underlying philosophy that guides the content of the rest of this book;

- Explore the advantages of reflection as a competency in frontline staff;

- Introduce readers to the model for structured reflection that will be used in the rest of this book.

WHAT IS REFLECTIVE PRACTICE?

Reflective practice can be defined as the process involved in making sense of events, situations, or actions that occur in practice settings; reflection, in this sense, emphasises a thoughtful approach to understanding experience, whether in real time or retrospectively (Boros, 2009, p. 23).

The origins of the concept of reflective practice can be found in the writings of the educationist and philosopher, John Dewey. Dewey described a way of making sense of experience which he termed 'reflective thought'. Reflective thought consists of the following elements:

- Developing a sense of the problem at hand

- Enriching that sense with observations of the relevant conditions

- Elaborating a conclusion

- Testing that conclusion in practice.

Reflective thinking serves to 'transform a situation in which there is obscurity, doubt, conflict, and disturbance of some sort, into a situation that is clear, coherent, settled, harmonious' (Dewey, 1933, pp. 101–102). Thinking reflectively makes the assumption that it is legitimate to approach situations with a flexible stance and modify our approach in the light of experience (Boros, 2009).

Dewey's ideas about the reflective process were further developed into a very widely used model of adult learning by David Kolb – we will consider this model further below. Contemporary thinking about the concept of reflective practice as it applies to professionals such as doctors, nurses, social workers and psychotherapists comes from the work of Donald Schön (1983) who formulated the key ideas of reflection-on-action and reflection-in-action in his book, *The Reflective Practitioner*.

Reflection-on-action

This kind of reflection is retrospective. Experiences, events and incidents are reviewed after they have occurred. We try to make sense of them through considering theories, guidelines, clinical experience, and our existing knowledge. The aim of reflection-on-action is to learn from the (recent) past in order to be better prepared for the future. An example of reflection-on-action is conducting a critical incident analysis on a hospital ward following a near miss or an accident (see *Chapter 2* for a detailed description of critical incident analysis).

Reflection-in-action

In this kind of reflection, we think on our feet. While engaged in practice, we use our existing knowledge and skills to modify our responses to the situation at hand in order to deal with it more effectively. An example of reflection-in-action is purposely managing your own reaction to a very angry service user at the doorstep so as not to aggravate the individual more and place yourself at risk of attack.

REFLECTIVE ACTIVITY

What do you think the benefits might be of the two kinds of reflective practice defined above (reflection-on-action and reflection-in-action) for yourself and your service?

Through developing a variety of reflective skills, practitioners empower themselves with tools for enhancing the efficiency with which they learn from their experiences. They enhance their responsiveness to the environment within which they operate and, ultimately, reflective practice should achieve better services for the public.

The rest of this chapter examines some of the mechanisms that underlie effective reflective practice and presents some of the benefits to services of developing their teams' capacity to reflect. We start by considering two complementary perspectives on adult learning, namely, the competence matrix and Kolb's experiential learning cycle.

THE COMPETENCE MATRIX

Think for a moment about a time when you had to learn a new skill; for instance, skiing, driving a car, or learning a new language. What was the process like? Learning something new often involves traversing the following four stages of skills acquisition, sometimes called the competence matrix (Gordon Training, date unknown). As you read the descriptions of the different stages, try to think of the process as you experienced it.

Stage 1: Unconsciously unskilled

People who are proficient at something make it look easy. In this first stage, we are almost unaware that we don't really know how to do it. This is especially the case if we are trying to master a variation on a skill we already possess, for instance, driving in another country. This can lead to a false sense of confidence in our ability that quickly disappears as we try our hand at it for the first time.

Stage 2: Consciously unskilled

In Stage 2, we are confronted with our initial inability as we try to learn. Our false confidence evaporates. 'I can do that!' becomes 'I wish I could do that', as we realise that the task ahead is daunting and we might need to start our learning on the bottom rung.

Stage 3: Consciously skilled

This stage represents the awkward early stage of the learning process where you are aware of every aspect of the skill you are trying to learn. A good example is the conscious thought processes which novice drivers often experience, where every step needed for a manoeuvre is rehearsed through internal dialogue. Over time, the awkwardness decreases as we become more fluent and the new skill starts to feel natural to us.

Stage 4: Unconsciously skilled

Stage 4 sets in when you stop thinking and just get on with things. You've mastered the skill and it becomes a natural extension of yourself. For example, you might just get in the car in the morning, set off, and the next thing you are aware of is that you arrive at work. You might have no awareness of consciously making many of the decisions regarding your driving that you had to make while on the way, for instance, about which gear to put the car in, or when to use the accelerator or the brake.

When you become experienced at your role, you may find yourself functioning in Stage 4. You might be more or less on autopilot most of the time and perform your various tasks fluently without too much of the step by step thinking that characterises the consciously skilled stage (and which makes it feel such a slow and awkward phase of the learning process).

What mature reflective practice does is to add a fifth phase to this process. Reflection takes you back to the consciously skilled phase *after* you've reached the unconsciously skilled stage. Reflection involves investing time and energy in thinking about and articulating what it is you are trying to achieve. You focus on becoming aware of how you approach the task at hand, what assumptions you are making in the process, how your own feelings and internal processes are affecting you, and how you can learn from these insights. All the while, you do not relinquish existing skills and you remain fluent at those aspects of your role you were able to perform fluently before. However, reflective practitioners become skilled at detecting and articulating their own reactions to their work and develop the problem solving tools and mental models to match their own processes with those of service users.

KOLB'S ADULT LEARNING CYCLE

David Kolb (1984) formulated a model of experiential learning that helps explain what happens during reflective learning when we engage with our experiences to learn from them. His theory was that adults learn through reflecting on observed reality and develop new concepts from these reflections. Reflective thought in this context refers to the ideas of Dewey, discussed earlier in this chapter. Once concept formation has taken place, actions are performed in the environment that test the newly formed concepts. The outcome of this 'testing phase' enables the concepts that were formed to be modified and the cycle starts again with observations on experience. Kolb devised a four-stage model of experiential learning that consists of the following stages:

Stage one: Observation

The first step of the experiential learning cycle involves observation. Learning starts with noticing things. Sometimes we learn profound lessons from everyday, mundane occurrences. For example, what is a service user's first encounter with your service like? Do they get a formal, official letter through the letter box? Do they have to face an imposing reception desk leading to a security-protected, reinforced door? Or do they receive a phone call from a friendly-sounding receptionist inviting them for an assessment appointment? As you might imagine, these different possibilities for an initial contact can lead to very different service user reactions to a service and may therefore explain a lot about service user engagement with services.

Noticing things involves two key personal attributes, curiosity and the ability to question assumptions that are generally taken for granted. The kind of assumptions I have in mind include both the assumptions that you bring into the workplace from your background and your life outside work, and the kind of assumptions that services make about the people who make use of their support, about other services, and about partner agencies. Most of the chapters that follow will invite you to articulate and critically question some of your own assumptions.

Questioning assumptions does not mean that those assumptions are necessarily wrong or unhelpful, but the process of bringing assumptions to the fore, naming them, and carefully considering their impact on the service, service users, and practitioners, allows practitioners to operate with more awareness of their own contribution to the outcomes they achieve and the difficulties they face.

Stages two and three: Reflection and concept development

Kolb's stages of reflection and concept development are highly interrelated phases in experiential learning and are key aspects of reflective practice, as defined in this book. Both of these steps involve making sense of experience. In order to reflect, you need self-awareness and self-knowledge. You need to be aware of how your own history, personality, and assumptions affect the way you provide services and how these attributes enable you to use yourself as a change agent.

Developing your reflective skills enables you to articulate and express how these internal processes come into play in your approach to your work. If you follow through on the cycle of experiential learning, this understanding can help you improve your practice.

The notion of concept development touches on another key aspect of the way in which reflective practice is interpreted in this book. Although developing an awareness of one's own assumptions and those of the service can be helpful in improving practice, practitioners can only be truly reflective in the way Dewey had in mind if they can make sense of and articulate their learning. Reflective practice is therefore inextricably bound to the language of reflection one chooses to use. In fact, there are three 'languages' involved in this process:

a) The first is your own professional language. As students, future practitioners acquire a vocabulary relevant to their respective practices: social workers learn the theories and terminology relevant to social work practice, childcare practitioners focus on child development theories, and nurses learn the language of anatomy, physiology, and nursing care.

b) The second language is that of self-awareness. Can you describe your own psychological processes? Are you able to identify and make sense of your own emotions, what the situations are that trigger these, and how you can effectively deal with your reactions to your professional experience? Can you express how you feel when demands on you are exceptionally high or when you feel bored and unstimulated at work? Are you aware of the times when you bring home life into work with you or when service users and their problems unhelpfully stay with you after work?

c) The third language is located between the first two: It is the language of the psychological process of service delivery. What words, concepts or theories can you use to make sense of service users' reactions to your efforts, their responses to you when you converse with them, the ways in which your service functions, and the ways in which service users approach the services you have on offer? How does your making sense of service user responses feed into the other systems in which they are embedded and how do these factors relate to you as a professional and as a person?

The different chapters in this book were written to help practitioners on their journeys toward developing these last two kinds of languages, the languages of self-reflection and of reflection on the work in frontline services. In this book, we are not concerned with the first kind of language, that of profession-specific theories and terminology, except insofar as some insights from the fields of psychology and psychodynamic theory provide very helpful perspectives on the human processes that practitioners are likely to encounter in the course of their work.

Stage four: Action

The fourth phase of Kolb's experiential learning cycle is about action and active experimentation. Reflective practice has little chance of enhancing service quality unless it leads to action and change in the real world. All of the following chapters contain practical exercises designed to influence your work practices. You can do these with your colleagues or on your own. However, in the final analysis it is up to you to invest your energy and enthusiasm to make change happen and improve practice.

Reflection that follows this four-stage cycle can happen in many ways and there are a number of models or structures that can be helpfully used as a guide to the reflective process. To help structure the way you practice reflection, we will follow a three-step framework throughout this book. It is a simplified form of Kolb's cycle discussed above, and consists of the following steps:

THE THREE-STEP (CLT) REFLECTIVE CYCLE

Step 1: Curiosity

As in the description of Kolb's learning cycle above, this step involves noticing things, asking questions, and questioning assumptions. This step enables practitioners to develop awareness of their own assumptions through astute observation and recognition of patterns where they occur.

Step 2: Looking closer

Zooming in on experiences, slowing down processes, and finding words that help to make sense of events or feelings fall within this stage. Openness to new perspectives is a prerequisite for successfully traversing this phase. Looking closer primarily involves finding a language to articulate the phenomena noticed in Step 1 and pressing home critical questions regarding accepted methods and individual or shared assumptions.

Step 3: Transformation and feedback

This phase is all about sense making and action. Using observations from the first step in conjunction with the insights gained from looking closer, the transformation phase is about finding ways to articulate content and process in a format that allows for positive changes to be made.

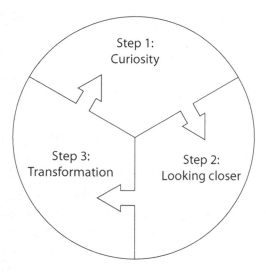

Figure 1.1 *The three-stage (CLT) model of reflection*

Examples of how this model of reflection can be implemented in practice are provided throughout this book. Readers who wish to take a quick detour to see how the CLT (Curiosity–Looking Closer–Transformation) model can be used for an effective, yet simple reflective process, can turn to *Chapter 2* where there is a worked example of CLT in action.

Achieving reflective practice in your service

There are a few prerequisites for achieving effective reflective practice within frontline services. Since reflective practice is about both individual development and the ways in which services are delivered, it would be very difficult for individual readers to be the sole reflective practitioners in their services. Individual enthusiasm should really be backed up by management and team 'buy-in'. Reflective practice works best if done in ways that combine individual and team effort. This means that organisations that commit to ensuring their staff are reflective practitioners also tend to commit to creating reflective spaces for their staff to develop their reflective skills. This involves making time and space available to individuals for reflection, and perhaps also offering opportunities for facilitated reflection in group contexts. The exercises in the rest of this book are designed to facilitate both of these kinds of reflection as they lend themselves to use in structured, facilitated groups as well as to use in individual reflection.

CHAPTER SUMMARY

Five key points to take away from Chapter 1:

- Reflective practice is a process that helps you make sense of your experiences at work.

- The ultimate aims of reflective practice are to improve practice and help practitioners deliver better services.

- Reflective practitioners can reflect on situations they encounter in the workplace both during the event (reflection-in-action) and after (reflection-on-action). Reflection can be practised alone, but is often most useful if done with others.

- Reflective practice enables practitioners to articulate those aspects of their practice they are 'unconsciously skilled' at, thus making their underlying assumptions explicit and increasing their ability to be accountable.

- A three-step cycle can be used to structure reflection: a stage of Curiosity where important questions are asked and assumptions questioned: a phase of Looking Closer at the experience through considering the questions asked in the initial step; and finally, a phase of Transformation, in which the results of Looking Closer are used to change perspectives and transform and improve practice.

FURTHER READING

There are a number of excellent introductory texts to the theory and practice of reflection in specific settings. If you would like to know more about reflective practice and its theoretical basis, the book by Donald Schön, *The Reflective Practitioner: How Professionals Think in Action*, is a good read as it is the source which most other authors on reflective practice tend to draw on. For applications to health care and nursing, Taylor (2006) is a good source, while social care practitioners could consult Knott & Scragg (2007).

02

HOW TO REFLECT: THE REFLECTIVE PRACTITIONER'S TOOLKIT

THIS CHAPTER AIMS TO:

- Consider how to create a reflective space through reflecting alone or with others;
- Introduce the benefits of using a reflective journal to record your learning;
- Equip you with practical tools for structured reflection;
- Provide examples of how to use the tools described in the text.

This chapter builds on the concept of reflective practice introduced in *Chapter 1*. We will take the CLT (Curiosity–Looking Closer–Transformation) framework for reflection used in the rest of this book, and add to this a toolkit of reflective techniques to help you develop both self-awareness and an understanding of the processes that might affect the lives of service users and the agencies who work with them. The techniques introduced range from very structured methods to more creative ways to express your experiences – all in the service of improving your skills as a reflective practitioner.

At first, the techniques you will learn about in this chapter, if practised regularly, will improve your ability to reflect on your work retrospectively (reflection-on-action in the Schön (1983) model). They will deepen your understanding of your own practice and enable you to look at all aspects of your practice from a different perspective and learn. In time, however, you should also become more skilled at reflection-in-action – taking a reflective stance in real time, while actively engaged in practice. With frequent practice, effective reflection should become second nature to you and permeate all aspects of your approach.

CREATING A REFLECTIVE SPACE

Reflecting alone or with others?

Although most of the practical techniques introduced in the next section can be done individually, you will almost certainly benefit from opportunities to reflect with others. This can take the form of jointly working through the chapters in this book with colleagues informally, or taking part in a facilitated reflective practice group. Group reflection brings with it a number of advantages, including:

• The ability to share similar experiences with colleagues;

• Benefiting from others' perspectives;

• Accessing mutual support;

• Opportunities to benefit from feedback from peers in a non-threatening setting;

• Opportunities for rehearsal, role play, and guided practice.

Individual reflection also has an important role to play in your development as a practitioner. You need time to think about and work though your personal reactions to the issues you come across in your work life. Individual reflection and a growing self-awareness combine with reflecting with others to help you develop your own thinking skills and enhance the extent to which you are 'present' in your role.

Making time for reflection

The importance of working at developing your reflective skills through individual and joint reflection alerts us to the need for making space for reflection in our work lives. Creating reflective space involves, first of all, making time for reflection in your busy schedule. In my experience, practitioners are prone to becoming so caught up in the pressures of their jobs that they find it difficult to find time for reflection. However, investing some of your precious work time in reflection can yield impressive gains not only in the quality of practice within teams, but also in the efficiency with which practitioners are able to complete their work. In other words, if you make time for reflective practice, you may find that you become more efficient rather than more pressurised in your role.

Creating reflective space also involves cultivating in yourself a reflective mindset which includes being open to new experiences and a readiness to learn. Learning in this context involves more than enhancing your technical knowledge and learning about new theories. The kind of learning that reflective practice will enhance includes knowing yourself better, acquiring a way to use yourself more effectively as a change agent to benefit service recipients, and developing ways of being with people that communicate empathy and understanding.

YOUR CORE TOOL FOR REFLECTION: THE REFLECTIVE JOURNAL

Keeping a reflective journal is generally seen as one of the most valuable tools in the reflective practitioner's toolkit (Ghaye, 2008; Ghaye & Lillyman, 2006; Jasper, 2003). There are many variations on the theme of the reflective journal, ranging from written journals and diaries to using blogs and social media. In my experience, a written journal in hard copy format can be a very useful tool for recording personal experiences, interactions and feelings about work-related issues. Writing in your journal regularly can foster a sense of immediacy and self-awareness regarding your own feelings about the experiences you encounter at work. It is also helpful for practice development to be able to review journal entries either in supervision or in structured, facilitated sessions for reflection. Having journal entries made over an extended period to look back on, can give you a sense of your professional and career development over time.

What do I write about?

The short answer to this question is anything that is relevant to the way the work you do relates to you as a person. You can record a wide range of practice stories, experiences and thinking processes, including:

- anecdotes;

- personal reactions to situations;

- things you have learned through practice, in supervision, in conversation with other professionals, whilst on training, or through personal study;

- your experiences of casework or what it is like to be part of the organisation you work for.

You can also use your journal as a creative space within which to experiment with different ways in which to conceptualise your work and to reflect on your role and how you understand it.

Many of the exercises in the rest of this book are also suited for use in reflective journals. The key to using your journal effectively is to make time to regularly write in it – even if only for 10 minutes a week. Establishing a habit of 'little and often' for journalling works well as this retains the sense of immediacy in the journal entries and allows you to reflect continuously on your experiences.

What can I gain from starting a reflective journal?

As mentioned above, you stand to gain very substantially from keeping a reflective journal. Procrastination and lack of time are the most frequently cited obstacles to starting and maintaining a reflective journal. Those practitioners who choose to make a small amount of time available for reflection on a regular basis, almost invariably report that the effort was very much worth their while.

Ghaye and Lillyman (2006) list some of the advantages their nursing students attributed to keeping reflective journals. These included the following:

- Journalling illuminated their thinking and showed them how open and receptive to new learning they were

- They were able to track how their thinking developed over time

- Journalling helped them to appreciate their general attitude towards their work

- Journalling helped them become better practitioners

- Keeping a journal motivated them and helped them in their advocacy role.

These are not insubstantial gains. Ghaye and Lillyman's list for nurses is certainly consistent with my experience in working with a range of practitioners across different settings.

Note on confidentiality:

If you decide to start a reflective journal, it is important that you give some thought to issues of confidentiality around your journal entries. Both your employer and your professional body may have some guidelines about confidentiality that you should follow. As a minimum measure, it would be very important to ensure that the identities of colleagues and service recipients should never be apparent from your journal entries.

You should also take great care to store your journal entries securely. If you are planning to use a reflective journal as part of a reflective practice group, it would be helpful if the group could reach some consensus on how confidentiality and anonymity would be protected within your journals. Similar considerations apply when any of the techniques discussed in this chapter are used in professional settings with confidential information.

Even if you ensure no one can be identified through your journal, you also need to know that, in the UK, under law, it is possible that your journal entries may be viewed as legal evidence and you may be required to release your entries to be entered into evidence in the Courts. However, the best way to ensure that your journalling is safe in this regard is to discuss the issues that keeping a journal raises for you in your setting with your line manager or course tutor.

An example of a journal entry

The following example of a journal entry uses the CLT framework given in *Chapter 1* to illustrate one practitioner's learning from an incident at work:

The most significant event at work yesterday was the phone call I had from social services in the morning. It stayed with me all day and I took the issue home with me which is not a good thing for my stress levels. They want to refer another child protection case to us. This time they have been involved with the family for years; the children have been on the child protection register for neglect and emotional abuse. When I asked what it was they wanted from our team, she asked us to go in and offer advice on boundaries and bedtime routine. But child and adolescent mental health services are involved and the family already has at least three other allocated workers from different agencies. I just felt so angry that they keep referring families with complex needs to us when we are a preventative service. The social worker was surprised when I asked her if she knew that we were a preventative service that only works with families for six weeks at a time. I told her she could complete a referral form for the team, but my heart had already sunk as I am sure we will end up carrying the case as we do in so many other instances. Why does this always happen to our team?

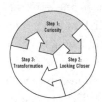

Curiosity

Why does this always happen to us? Do we as a team ever say 'no' to referrals? Do other people know that we are only a preventative service? Why am I so upset when this happens?

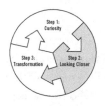

Looking closer

I thought about this incident all night and came to the conclusion that we as practitioners – and that includes me – have created a culture amongst ourselves of not saying 'no' to work coming in; we hold on to families, perhaps thinking we can rescue them. Usually the discussion in team meetings or in supervision goes something like 'If I don't stay involved with them, no one will be there to support (or rescue) them, or social services will do nothing.' Is this really true?

I also don't think we as a team have agreed and written down referral criteria, so referrers don't know what we can and cannot offer.

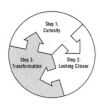

Transformation

I will start to listen more closely to myself and my colleagues when we talk with each other about the people we work with to see if we are really 'rescuers' and what that means for us personally and for our practice. It might also be good to raise the questions about saying 'no' to referrals and discharging people a little quicker at team meetings.

This morning I suggested to my colleague who was in early with me, that we do an information leaflet on our service and she agreed that that was a great idea, so we will raise this with our manager.

This example of a journal entry illustrates several aspects of the learning that can be done through reflective journalling. First of all it illustrates that any practitioner open to reflective practices can use structured reflective techniques to learn from their experiences. The example chosen shows a common dilemma in services where there are conflicts between demands and needs and how these are reflected in the interrelationships between different agencies – and how these relationships can impact on the work lives of individual practitioners. It also illustrates how individual and joint action can result from reflecting on work-based situations.

Using a structured guideline, such as the CLT model of reflection, is just one way this practitioner could have used her journal to reflect on this situation. The CLT model guides you through the reflective process, ensuring that you invest time and effort in trying to come to an understanding of the practice situation that you are reflecting upon. It also directs your thinking to the ways in which reflection helps you to transform your approach to your practice and improve the way you work. Alternative approaches to journal reflection include using techniques such as illuminative incident analysis or critical incident analysis, both of which are described below.

Finally, the above example illustrates that reflection is an ongoing process. The practitioner concerned may engage in further reflection cycles as she follows up the ideas generated by her first reflective cycle. At a later date she might reflect on further developments within her team regarding their response to her idea that they may not be clear on who they accept or reject to their service. As such, any one reflective cycle can be followed up by further reflection that extends and elaborates on developments over time. This ongoing, continuous process of reflection is what characterises reflective practice as an approach to continuous professional development.

Interspersed between different sections of this book, there are four extended examples that elaborate and develop the idea of journal-based reflection for readers. These illustrate further examples of the CLT framework for structured reflection. But there are also other reflective methods illustrated in the examples. Through providing these, I hope that you will find inspiration in using reflective techniques to help you develop your own reflective skills and improve your service.

Levels of reflection

Goodman (1984) identifies three levels of reflection, two of which are illustrated in the previous example of a journal entry. The first level of reflection involves accurate description

– identifying the salient features of a situation you wish to reflect on. In the example above, the practitioner identified both personal reactions to events and features of those events as suitable material for reflection. At this level, awareness of one's own reactions to events is very important. For example, the practitioner in the example identified that the enquiry about a possible new referral that came in triggered stress and worry for her that impacted on her life outside work. It also brought to the fore a growing realisation of possible personal and team dynamics around rescuing others and feeling burdened with caring for vulnerable service users, despite this not being the core purpose of the service. At this level, an understanding of individual and team dynamics from the various perspectives covered in this book can equip practitioners with the thinking tools to reflect effectively.

The second level of reflection involves drawing conclusions from observations and coming up with solutions that improve services or address the problems that came to light during the reflective process. Increased practitioner insight in personal or collective practice – such as the suggestions for transformation mentioned in the example – can deliver tangible benefits for services, but also provide the root material for further reflection. In the given example, practitioners' tendencies toward being rescuers was one of the phenomena that aroused curiosity – practitioners may wish to explore such phenomena further using structured reflective tools such as Johari's window, discussed below.

It is also helpful to appreciate that the example illustrates the tentative and unfinished nature of any one 'episode' of reflection – suggested changes may need further reflection and evaluation after implementation; personal reactions may need follow-up and discussion in supervision; and team or organisational changes may bring to light further issues that elicit reflection. The reflective process is therefore an open-ended exploration of the boundary between the personal and professional.

The third level of reflection involves appreciating the wider social, political and societal influences that come into play within the incident or situation that is the focus of reflection. In the example above, the practitioner showed some awareness of inter-agency pressures and the impact of these on other agencies (social services in this instance), but did not focus her reflective process on exploring these issues for her service. In contemporary service settings, this level of reflection is likely to touch frequently on the many conflicts between resources and needs that affect service delivery on the front line in the modern welfare state.

A selection of tools for structured reflection

The reflective tools discussed in this section are offered as structured techniques that might help you to reflect on specific situations or cases you come across. They are mostly aimed at enhancing understanding of complex situations and issues that practitioners often encounter. Most of these can be done either individually or in group settings. Some of them will be illustrated in more depth in the four extended worked examples that are provided throughout this book.

Mapping out self-understanding – a variation on Johari's window

How does your personality affect your approach to work? How do others perceive you? How open are you to learning about new ideas that can enhance your practice? What if those ideas involve facing up to the many different sides of who you are? And what if you come face to face with how others perceive you in the process?

Self-awareness is a key element of reflective practice as the term is used in this book. Understanding our own processes and how these influence the way in which we approach our work can help us to use ourselves more effectively as change agents. One very helpful tool to support self-exploration is called Johari's window. It is named after Joseph Luft and Harry Ingham, two psychologists who invented the technique in the 1950s.

The idea behind Johari's window is fairly simple; namely, that there are some things about us that are known only to us, while there are also things about us that others may notice even though we are unaware of them (Luft & Ingham, 1955). In between these extremes are personality traits that both we and others are aware of. The Johari's window system is completed by considering those aspects of our functioning that are as yet unconscious – unknown to ourselves and to others. These unknown elements of our personalities may be those areas of our functioning that have never been elicited due to our never being exposed to the circumstances that would bring these traits to the fore. The four combinations can be represented as a two-by-two grid, as illustrated below.

Table 2.1 *The four quadrants of Johari's window*

	Known to **others**	Unknown to **others**
Known to **self**	**Open**	**Hidden**
Unknown to **self**	**Blind**	**Unknown**

Looking at the quadrants of Johari's window in turn:

- The **open** area represents things known about you to yourself, as well as to others.

- The **hidden** area represents aspects of your personality known to you, but not to others.

- The **blind area** is known to others, but you are unaware of these perceptions of you.

- The **unknown** area represents those elements of your functioning that are unknown both to yourself and to others.

Through becoming more reflective in your practice, your open quadrant will tend to expand. You may start to understand and recognise elements of yourself that you bring into work that you were previously unaware of, especially through eliciting feedback from others (thus shrinking the blind quadrant). You may also find ways to share and explore elements of yourself with others which you previously hung on to, perhaps for fear of looking incompetent, unprofessional, or perhaps unworthy. Through self-disclosure the hidden quadrant becomes smaller, and the open area expands.

Over time, you might find that unknown aspects of your response to your work practice reveal themselves to you, perhaps in unexpected ways. You might just be able to capture these elusive revelations before they disappear from your awareness and record them using the Johari grid. Bringing these aspects of yourself into the light is a key step towards integrating them into your self-awareness.

Please note that all of us will always have all four of these quadrants – and it is not desirable to eliminate any of them completely from our personalities. However, as you become more reflective you may become more able to reduce your **blind** area by requesting feedback from others, reduce your **hidden area** by developing skills at appropriate self-disclosure, and reduce your **unknown area** through a process of self-discovery, and processing others' observations of you.

The original Johari's window technique involved using adjective checklists to complete the four quadrants, but this is not the only way one can use the grid. Reflective practitioners may decide to include a Johari's window framework in their journals and, where relevant, indicate on the grid where aspects of their practice fall during the times they use their journals for reflection.

Johari's window is a useful tool in supporting the process of working with hidden and blind spots to foster greater self-understanding, but it also reminds us that there are elements of not seeing and not knowing that are always present in the work. These unknown, unpredictable, perhaps even impenetrable elements of work in frontline services are always in the background and can be the source of considerable anxiety in practitioners. Awareness of the existence and contents of such hidden sides of our personalities can help us to understand and accept even the shadow sides of ourselves as practitioners and consequently lead to improved self-insight. The benefit to services lies in the enhancement of their capacity to match service needs with practitioners who are best suited to meet these.

Example of how to use Johari's window:

Joanne is a family support practitioner who was sent on a residential training course on attachment theory and working with vulnerable families. The training was both theoretical and experiential. She used Johari's window to capture some of her experiential learning on the training course:

Table 2.2 *Example of a completed Johari's window*

	Known to **others**	Unknown to **others**
Known to **self**	**Open** Bubbly & enthusiastic about new ideas; Enjoys doing things more than thinking about theories; Very moved by vulnerable children and their plight; Gets stressed easily.	**Hidden** Feels very vulnerable when confronted with strong personalities; Confidence is a sham – full of doubts regarding own abilities; Worried about small things in relationships – will they still love me if they find out who I am? Own history of insecure attachment carefully kept a secret.
Unknown to **self**	**Blind** Tremendous empathy with vulnerable people and respecting of their choices and actions; Can get very angry if feeling rejected; Works very hard at being accepted by everyone; Takes on 'mothering'/caring role.	**Unknown** Brief moments of very strong anxious feelings never experienced before.

Joanne's learning about herself involved realisations moving from the blind and unknown sections of Johari's window into her open and hidden areas during the course of her residential week. This happened as she became more aware of those aspects of herself through interacting with the other participants and the course facilitators. She used Johari's window to summarise where, in her view, the different elements of her personality resided before she become aware of them.

Taking a closer look at the hidden elements, she might decide to become more open in supervision about her feelings of vulnerability and her lack of confidence. She may still decide not to share her insecure attachment history with others. She might have been surprised to learn that others viewed her as hard working, very caring, and empathic. Perhaps the intensity of her anger and the depth of her anxiety may also have been surprising to her. Learning in this way from her own experience and the feedback from others may enable her to understand herself more fully and manage her reactions to work situations better.

Finally, the hidden feelings of deep anxiety may relate to her attachment history. At any one point in time hidden aspects of our personalities may only partially reveal themselves to us. It is not essential to unearth these completely, but over time Joanne might experience more clarity on the significance of these feelings and how they affect her in her work and personal lives.

It is likely that Joanne only shared a part of her learning about herself with others, but the Johari's window exercise helped her capture what she had learnt and enabled her to think about how her experiential learning can help her in her role.

Thinking about critical incidents: critical incident analysis

Originally, critical incident analysis was developed in the aviation industry to analyse effective and ineffective behaviour in certain situations. In health care practice, these techniques have become very widely used, primarily to help practitioners think about situations where something did not quite go according to plan; for example, drug errors and other reportable incidents. Ghaye and Lillyman (2006) point out that critical incident analysis can be a very useful methodology for practitioners who are interested in reflecting on their experiences with the purpose of experiential learning: An incident becomes a 'critical incident' once it is the focus of reflection and learning. Thus ordinary experiences from daily practice as well as extraordinary experiences such as near misses can be used as the basis for a critical incident analysis.

Tripp (1993) suggests that we can approach critical incidents in the following ways:

First of all, we should ask ourselves questions both about what actually took place, and what did not happen. Asking ourselves questions about 'non-events' can lead to powerful learning and improvements in practice.

The second method he talks about is the 'why?' challenge. Delving deeper into the reasons why we engage in certain actions may lead us to the roots of our assumptions. Very often the answer to the question 'why?' is 'because that is the way we have always worked'. There may be a rich history behind embedded practice routines, but that does not guarantee a sound evidence base or clinical effectiveness. One of the aims of reflective practice is to question deeply held assumptions with regard to frontline practice in order to give practitioners the tools with which to effect positive change at all levels.

The third method Tripp suggests is to identify dilemmas inherent in the incident. What are the aspects of the situation within which you feel caught between two difficult alternatives? How did you resolve the dilemmas you faced? Is there a different or better way to achieve resolution than the one you followed?

Fourthly, we need to make explicit our own personal theories regarding the incident and the people involved. Which of your values informed the way you managed the incident and how did that affect your work and your approach?

Lastly, critical incidents should be located within their broader social and political contexts, an idea very similar to the third level of reflection mentioned earlier (Goodman, 1984). Which ideological assumptions did you make in your approach to the situation? Would you have acted differently if you operated from a different ideological stance? Although our underlying assumptions are often very difficult to identify and articulate, they are important in explaining our behaviour in many situations and can be at the root of acting in ways that we might ourselves find difficult to understand. Examples of ideological assumptions include the ways in which you characterise the people who use your service, how your political views affect your practice, and how you respond to current government policies that affect your area of practice.

Ghaye and Lillyman (2006) offer a slightly simpler framework for recording critical incidents. They suggest that you cover the following aspects of each incident:

- What happened? (description of the incident)

- Who was involved?

- What were the outcomes of the incident?

- What did I/they learn?

- How did this incident affect my practice?

The following example from the journal of a practitioner in a children's home embeds this framework within the CLT model for reflection discussed in *Chapter 1*.

Last Friday afternoon Lennie ran out into the road again. He had an argument with one of the other care staff shortly before and became very aggressive towards all of the staff afterwards. Because of his behaviour he lost some of his privileges for the weekend. I observed all this, but was not involved in any of the altercations and was able to spend some one to one time with him. Yet I left work somehow feeling that we had failed him.

Who was involved?

Thinking back, apart from Lennie, there were two other male carers and myself. The other males are generally more assertive and robust with the young people, while I tend to be quieter and keep to the background when there are confrontations.

Who did what?

Lennie was originally upset because Steve would not let him go to the shops on his own. Lennie argued that Steve allowed two of the other young people to go on their own, so why couldn't he? He would not accept any explanation or reason and became more and more upset. Steve responded by raising his voice and telling Lennie that was the end of it, no further discussion was to be had. Lennie stormed off towards the front door, and went out into the road. Steve and Martin followed him and forcibly brought him back in as he wanted to go out in front of the cars. Lennie became very distressed and had to be restrained. I saw all of this from the hallway.

Once he was restrained, Lennie started crying, saying he is always treated like a baby and no one trusts him. After he had calmed down, I spent some one to one time with him. Martin hurt his hand during the restraint and was in the office trying to sort that out. When Lennie and I sat talking, he kept telling me about his mum and dad and how his dad was always violent towards her and that he used to hide behind the sofa when his dad came home drunk.

Learning

I finished my shift with a sense that we had failed Lennie and wanted to reflect more on this in my journal. Something in me was very ill at ease with the whole episode. Steve and Martin documented the whole thing, but when I read what they wrote before I left work, I felt that the team's account was a little bit one-sided and did not take Lennie's feelings into account, only his actions.

The care worker went on to use the CLT framework to further his reflections on the incident:

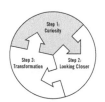

Curiosity

I have so many questions about this afternoon. What was it in the situation that made me feel we had failed Lennie? On reflection, I often feel this about our work with the young people. What was it about us that brought out his anger and aggression? What was my response about this – he never confronted me, and I never confronted him – was I the only one not involved? What do I feel about him? What is it about confrontation I don't like – or is that an issue at all?

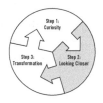

Looking closer

Reading Lennie's file, I noticed that he came from a family where there was a lot of domestic violence, alcohol and drug use, but he also had numerous failed placements. It's like when he hit 10 years of age, he spun out of control. So there are issues for him of boundaries, attachment and feeling that he can't be controlled and contained in a placement – and all the messages to him so far have been about not being manageable when this side of him came out: 'You are too aggressive, move on to the next, more restrictive place.' People are already thinking he is in line for a secure unit or an out of county placement. What does Lennie do when he feels upset – lash out or place himself in danger as if to say, 'I need you to be able to care for me when I attack you like I was attacked/in danger or when I place myself in danger'?

There is also another serious question. How do we as a team respond to Lennie? We all like him, but then we become very punitive towards him and despairing when he loses control. It's as if we lose control as well and Lennie and our feelings about him become unmanageable all at the same time.

But what about me? I think I know now that I am more an observer than an active participant when strong emotion and confrontation happens. This has never been an issue for me before, but I guess it's to do with some of my memories when Dad raised his voice when I was a child. Never liked confrontation – so I withdraw. I wonder how – and if – I can use this to help Lennie?

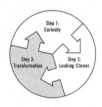

Transformation

It's important that I raise the issue of our reactions reflecting Lennie's emotions in the team meeting tomorrow. I will also take to supervision what I learned about myself. Perhaps I'm not assertive in other situations as well – so maybe I should get some feedback and do something about this. It's almost certain that I will get involved in some kind of confrontation sooner or later while I am doing this job so I might as well start working on becoming more comfortable with confrontation.

It is also interesting to see first hand how society, i.e. us as a home and the social services, respond to young people like Lennie who are 'out of control' with ever stronger attempts to restrict them which then only leads to them failing in many different contexts. It's so sad for me to see this in action. I wonder how we as a team can prevent this from happening for Lennie in our service, or even if we can?

A process such as that described here would take place over a number of days and, like most episodes of reflection, it is likely to raise a number of important questions that might not be answerable at the time. The process is also almost always incomplete, but raises questions that can form the focus of further reflection. However, practitioners benefit in many ways. They may gain enhanced insight into their own functioning as individuals within the workplace, increased sensitivity to both specific issues relating to their individual settings and broader issues that reside within the system as a whole, and helpful ideas their teams could take on board to improve practice.

Drawing things out: illuminative incident analysis

As mentioned in *Chapter 1*, the work in frontline settings can often be fraught with strong emotions in everyone involved. When an incident occurs within such a loaded context, there is often a lot of pressure on teams to come up with the causes and to identify who is to blame. In multi-agency work, it is rare to find individual agencies not pointing the finger at other agencies: 'This would never have happened if the social worker had done her job properly.' 'It is the nurse who should have noticed the signs of the problem and alerted the rest of us.' 'I can't believe the foster carers did not report the problem.'

Illuminative incident analysis was developed by Cortazzi and Roote in the 1970s as a way to help teams come to an understanding of the many factors involved in incidents and move forward in new ways with the lessons learnt (Cortazzi & Roote, 1975). Illuminative incident analysis involves using a series of visual representations such as group drawings and cartoons to depict an incident from different perspectives and learn from this what happened in the context of a strict rule of 'no blame'. They cite a number of examples where teams using this method in health care settings with people with intellectual disabilities managed to work through serious failures in care to find solutions that brought extended teams together and led to better care of patients.

Originally, this technique involved a facilitated group process, but the basic technique can be adapted for individual use. As an exercise to see how this might work for you, try the following:

REFLECTIVE ACTIVITY

Make a drawing that shows yourself and how you feel in relation to work right now. The artistic quality of what you draw is not important, but try to find a way to show your relationships to the different factors that affect your work life.

The following example (*Figure 2.1*, overleaf) links back to the reflective episode regarding the social services referral described earlier and illustrates how this method can help to foster understanding of a complex situation.

In order to get the most out of using illuminative incident analysis, you may find it helpful to make a series of drawings from the perspective of several of the parties involved in the incident you want to reflect on. You may also want to ask yourself questions such as 'Where is the service user in all of this?' (Cortazzi & Roote, 1975).

Capturing history: time lines

Time lines have been used in psychotherapy for many years now and have become a key tool in many psychological approaches. Usually a time line consists of a graph where the horizontal axis represents the passage of time, indicated either through chronological markers (years/months/ages) or through significant events. The height of the graph indicates the variable of concern which can be, for example, level of engagement with work, how much you enjoyed your role, or degree of job stress. Time lines can be constructed for many purposes, including:

- Mapping out critical incidents
- Visually representing your career development
- Correlating life events with career events.

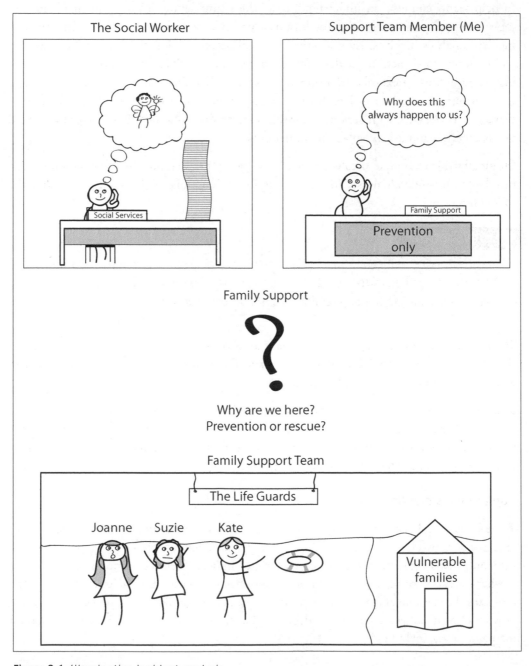

Figure 2.1 *Illuminative incident analysis*

The following example illustrates how a time line can be used to help understand how someone came to be where they are in their work life:

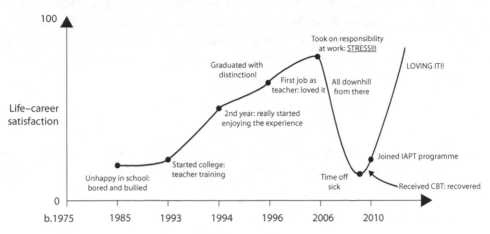

Figure 2.2 *Career time line: Haseen, an IAPT worker*

The reflective conversation: talking with a 'critical friend'

Beverley Taylor, in her introduction to reflective practice for nurses and midwives, introduces the helpful idea of a conversation with a 'critical friend' (Taylor, 2006). A critical friend is someone whom you choose to support your reflective practice; their role is to listen to your practice stories and ask you questions that are geared towards helping you reflect critically on your practice. The role of the critical friend is not to criticise you, but to support you in looking at your practice in ways that help you to identify your blind spots and learn from your experience.

Critical friend conversations centre around practice stories and the role of the critical friend might be to ask questions such as the following:

• What happened?

• Who was involved?

• What was your role?

• How did you feel when...?

• How do you explain the situation to yourself?

• What alternative views/options were there in the situation?

Although Taylor's original concept involves asking a colleague to be your critical friend, you could also use a group of colleagues to be critical friends, or even try to have a 'critical friend' dialogue with yourself in your journal, as the following fictional example dialogue illustrates:

Self: The family I visited yesterday. The mum has three children and she just lets them run riot in the house. It's such a mess. They are so demanding and she just sat there ignoring everything around her. Even talking to her was a chore as she answered questions with only the most basic information. I was so frustrated when I left, I just wanted to wake her up and get her to have a bit of energy.

Critical friend: So what do you think was happening for her? And for you?

Self: Thinking about it, I guess she felt overwhelmed. She is quite isolated and the kids are very demanding. Her partner is away most of the week and she might be depressed. But she is not keeping even basic standards of cleanliness and the kids need boundaries which she is just not putting in place.

Critical friend: What about you?

Self: I felt angry and impatient with her, I just want her to pull her socks up and start cleaning the place and teaching the children some discipline. I guess I'm action orientated and always felt that people should really attack problems actively rather than waiting for something to happen to resolve things. I know it might be a serious bout of depression, but I never had much sympathy with people who just give up.

Critical friend: How is your reaction going to help or hinder her?

Self: Perhaps my anger and impatience is similar to what she gets from her partner. I left with the feeling that he could be around more if he wanted to but that he withdrew from the family because of how she is. So I guess I'm not helping things to move forward much. I suggested counselling for her depressed feelings but she has the kids and no childcare which means she cannot attend appointments. Perhaps we can do something about that. She also said that she is conscious of being overweight and afraid of using public transport in case people stare at her. Perhaps my attitude could make her feel more judged.

Critical friend: What would a better situation look like?

Self: I would just like to see her get out of the house a little more – perhaps access a group or two for the kids and address the hygiene factors in the home. If she did a course on cooking healthy foods at the children's centre where there is a crèche and maybe we can find some funding to put a cleaner in for a one-off clean of the place, that might help. I could also talk to our support worker who works with dads, perhaps she can get dad to be a little more involved.

Critical friend: How do you feel now?

Self: I am still keen that she starts to help herself, but if she feels overwhelmed by the children and the house with no support, then perhaps we can help her in small ways to get there. It is a start. Maybe I'm not quite so impatient now.

In this example, an imaginary critical friend conversation gave the practitioner permission to question her own assumptions and to move on in the way she felt about a family and her work with the mum. Many issues remained unresolved, but the exercise allowed for a way forward to be found and the practitioner could explore both her empathic and impatient selves.

Engaging your creative side: music, movement, poetry and prose as reflection

As we have seen in the previous chapter, reflecting on practice involves making sense of our experiences at work. Since experience involves all of the senses, reflecting can involve all of the modalities of expression, including creative arts (Jasper, 2003; Lillyman & Ghaye, 2006; Taylor, 2006). Writing a poem that expresses your feelings about a certain incident, using prose or even music or movement (dance) to express your experience and make sense of it in a different way can assist you in developing your self-awareness as a practitioner.

REFLECTIVE ACTIVITY

Can you turn the picture below into a story that reflects the way your service operates?

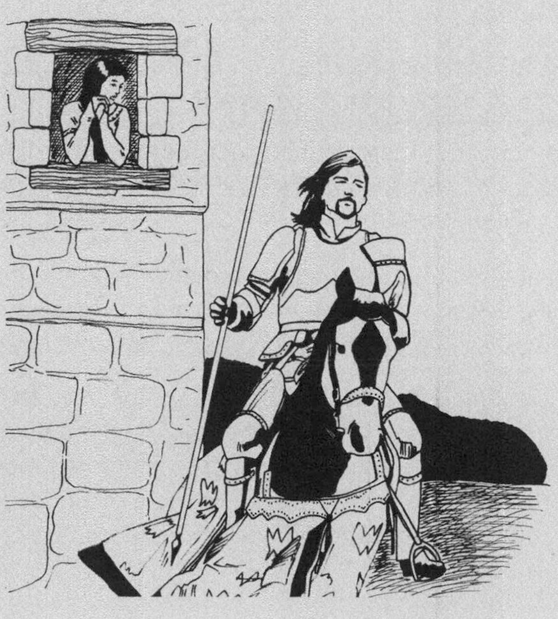

Figure 2.3 *A valiant knight to the rescue: how does this apply to your service?*

Here are some further examples of exercises that you can do alone or with your team to explore the creative side of reflection:

• Retell a practice story as a fairy tale, e.g. Little Red Riding Hood. What roles in the story would be taken up by professionals from the different agencies involved and which would be taken up by a service user? How can the ways in which the different characters interact be changed to improve the outcome – and how does that translate back into actions you can take to improve the service?

• Ask each team member to try to write a limerick that captures your role. How does yours compare with those of your colleagues? What are the important learning points from this exercise that you can take forward as a team?

• When you next discuss a complex case or a practice dilemma, ask your colleagues to be characters in the story and place them as sculptures around the room. What can you learn from each one's feedback on what it was like for them to be placed in the positions you asked them to take? What are the implications for you regarding this specific case?

CHAPTER SUMMARY

Five key points to take away from Chapter 2:

⊶ In order to reflect effectively, you need to create a reflective space for yourself. This may involve taking time out from other pressures to engage in reflective activities.

⊶ It is often helpful to reflect together with others in a facilitated group, although reflecting alone can also be effective.

⊶ Any work experiences are legitimate objects of reflection. Often the mundane aspects of work life can provide helpful insights that are useful in transforming services.

⊶ Techniques that can be used for structured and unstructured reflection include keeping a journal, making images, group work, and more creative activities such as writing poetry, making music or constructing role plays.

⊶ This chapter presented a range of tools that can be used to foster self-understanding and an understanding of service users' perspectives. These include Johari's window, illuminative incident analysis, time lines, 'critical friend' conversations and the CLT reflective cycle mentioned in *Chapter 1*. Examples of how to use these techniques for reflective practice are presented throughout this book.

FURTHER READING

This chapter introduced you to a number of techniques you can fruitfully use to enhance your ability to reflect in structured and creative ways on your practice. The books by Jasper (2003) and Taylor (2006) provide many excellent examples of additional reflective methods specific to nursing and health care. Ghaye and Lillyman (2006) offer detailed guidance on critical incident analysis and learning journals. Throughout the text of this book, there are also many other worked examples of reflective journal entries and further illustrations of some of the other techniques introduced in this chapter.

PART TWO

REFLECTING ON THE WORK IN FRONTLINE SERVICES

03

WORKING WITH PEOPLE'S STORIES: THE ROLE OF NARRATIVE IN FRONTLINE PRACTICE

THIS CHAPTER AIMS TO:

- Help you understand how narratives surround us in everyday life as well as in our professional lives;

- Help you reflect on the social functions of narratives such as folk tales and fairy tales;

- Help you consider how various narratives permeate practice in frontline services;

- Help you find ways to use insights from narrative approaches in everyday practice.

We live our lives surrounded by stories. From the fairy tales of childhood, to the ways in which events are reported in the news media, narratives of many sorts permeate our lives.

In fact, humans are inherently predisposed to develop ways of making meaning and, for the most part, accomplish this through constructing narratives: oral histories, religious narratives and folk tales are all forms of story that recount aspects of the human condition, people's experience of living in certain contexts, and the cultural wisdom that is handed down through the generations. Our collective memory as a human race is largely contained in stories that we tell in our various histories and cultures. This chapter argues that frontline practice is also permeated by narratives. It will explore this dimension of the work, focusing on narratives around services, service users and the human needs that are addressed within frontline settings.

THE SOCIAL FUNCTION OF MYTHS AND FOLK TALES

Stories have been part of human culture from very early on in the existence of the human race. For example, very early cave paintings contain narrative elements such as depictions of hunting or religious ceremonies. Ancient civilisations (and modern ones for that matter) went to great lengths to record and preserve accounts of their achievements. Folk tales and myths have been part of our oral traditions for thousands of years – and these ancient stories are still being told to children the world over. They have an appeal that transcends time. Well-known stories such as Little Red Riding Hood and Sleeping Beauty came into existence many centuries before their 'Disneyfication'. One of the reasons for their wide appeal throughout the ages is that they tend to reflect universal aspects of human experience. For instance, many fairy tales have themes that are relevant to children's experiences of growing up:

• Relationships with parents and step-parents

• Anxieties over 'What is to become of me?'

• Finding a sense of belonging

• Overcoming immense odds

• Going on a journey of discovery

• Violent fantasies and fears of destruction, annihilation, and engulfment (e.g. Hansel and Gretel)

• Themes of justice and revenge.

Folk tales illustrate the idea of growth and transformation through successfully dealing with suffering, pain and distress. They give an account of origins, create a shared belief system, and answer important questions about life in a way that makes sense, given the imagination and fantasy world of their audiences. Folk tales create a sense of certainty and resolution where there is uncertainty, fear and difficult dilemmas (Kast, 1995).

You may even find that some people feel that their lives reflect some of the myths and stories in our heritage. Do you know a Sisyphus who always tries extremely hard, only to find that disaster strikes just as success is about to come? Sisyphus offended the gods and his eternal punishment was to push a heavy boulder up a steep hill, only for the boulder to roll back down the hill every time he was about to accomplish the task, thereby forcing him to start again. How about a 'Little Red Riding Hood' who is constantly hoodwinked by a 'wolf in grandma's clothing', i.e. someone pretending to be safe?

Although these examples may be amusing, it is also true that a surprisingly large number of people can give a rather precise answer to the question, 'What happens to someone like me?' The reason for this lies in the way in which relationship and other patterns tend to repeat themselves in our lives. For instance, how do you achieve success? Through planned, structured effort, or by 'flying by the seat of your pants'? Do you view yourself as someone who always has bad luck, or are you the envy of your friends because you are so lucky? In recognising these repeating patterns in our lives, we are able to gain clues about which narrative strands we have used to construct our life stories. Practitioners of narrative therapies believe that, once we have recognised these patterns, we are able to address them and re-author our lives. This involves engaging with people's personal narratives, often in gentle but playful ways, as the following exercise illustrates. (This book contains several chapters that invite you to consider repeating patterns in people's lives from different angles: Two examples are in *Chapters 4* and *5*. *Chapter 4* looks at how attachment patterns that originate in childhood can lead to repeating patterns in dependency relationships in people's lives through the action of their internal working models. *Chapter 5* considers the impact of family history and inter-generational transmission of behavioural patterns.)

REFLECTIVE ACTIVITY

Take one of your favourite fairy tales and try to imagine how the tale would be different if told from a different vantage point or if one or more of the details were changed. Retell the story using a different main character, a different setting, or a different ending. Examples you could try include: retelling Little Red Riding Hood as a Western, or from the viewpoint of the wolf, Hansel and Gretel from the viewpoint of the wicked witch, or Snow White from the perspective of one of the dwarfs. While you are doing this exercise, try to become aware of the natural direction in which the narrative unfolds, given the new perspective you apply to it. Does the story feel right if you keep all the events and characters exactly as in the original, or is there another direction that feels more natural?

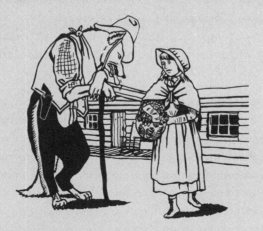

Figure 3.1 *How would the well-known tale of 'Little Red Riding Hood' be different if told from a new perspective?*

1. How do the ways in which the different characters in the story are portrayed differ between your version and the traditional version of the story?

2. How do the differences in viewpoint affect the way in which different events are construed within your story? Would you say that your alternative viewpoint still leaves you comfortable with the traditional ending of the story, or would the narrative lead to a different natural conclusion in your version?

3. Can you see applications of such a playful approach to story within the way you support service users? What, if anything, did you learn about your role as a practitioner from doing this exercise?

NARRATIVES IN FRONTLINE SETTINGS

As practitioners in frontline services, you have the rare privilege to be part of the cast of characters that form the stories of children, families or people in need who use your service. You have a role in helping them construct and reconstruct their lives. The ways in which you are able to do this will differ from service to service: therapists might be able to help people become more aware of the stories they live and help them re-author these directly. In family support services, the space to explain themselves might be liberating for parents of children in need, as would practical, concrete help to make things better. Many a fairy tale contains a benign helper who makes things better by magic. If you are the conduit to the resources that can improve a family's quality of life, you are a practitioner of a kind of 'magic'.

Teachers and classroom support staff have a more direct impact on the stories of children themselves. However, just through even cursory contact with the main adults in children's lives, they may be able to tell much of a child's experience of the world through observing interactions with carers at important times of transition: for example, when children are dropped off at school, when they are collected, and when carers interact with them during these times.

In your work with service users, what are the various kinds of 'story' you encounter? There are many aspects of frontline services where the work can be conceptualised as narratives. For example, referrals into a service represent stories of why someone or some group of people needs the service on offer. During assessments, service users construct narrative accounts of their lives, their problems, and their expectations of services or of practitioners, as well as the outcomes they hope for from their involvement. Professionals create narratives about the response of users to their service and different agencies have stories about each other. As we shall see in the chapter on supervision (*Chapter 12*), supervising the work that takes place in frontline settings involves working with several intersecting layers of narrative, including supervisees' narratives of their work, their organisation, partner agencies and the supervisor.

At the same time, supervisors have narratives about supervision, service users, their own agencies, and partner agencies. It is therefore vital that you remain aware of how you and your service construct the stories of the people you work with. For example, in professional settings, there is a danger for service users to be constructed in terms of pathologising discourses. Examples of this include diagnostic labels or administrative categories. This can blind practitioners and support staff to the individuality and uniqueness of people and the richness of each person's subjective experiences and needs.

It is also important to remain aware that reflective practice is all about stories and storytelling. Reflection takes place at the junction between your story, the stories of those you support, and the agencies who work with them. Creating and recreating stories is a powerful way to think about your work. The next exercise invites you to explore this idea further.

REFLECTIVE ACTIVITY

If you were to depict your service and your role within it as a fairy tale, fable or myth, what would that story be? How would it start, what would the plot be, and how would it end? What would you call the story?

The journalling exercise for this chapter is to write down your own version of this story and make a visual representation to illustrate it. If you are working through this chapter in a group of colleagues from your own team, it would be interesting to join forces and create a joint team story to which everyone contributes. Take your story to a team meeting and reflect on your own and your colleagues' reactions to it. What did you as a team learn from this that has implications for your practice?

NARRATIVE PRACTICE IN FRONTLINE SETTINGS

One very powerful way in which an understanding of people's stories can positively impact on practice in frontline services, is through applying some of the principles of narrative therapy. Narrative therapy is a relatively recent development in the field of family and systemic therapy (Sween, 1998; White, 2007). The fundamental assumption of narrative therapy is that many human problems are socially constructed and maintained in people's lives through dominant and oppressive narratives, while individual strengths and resilience can often be found by enabling people to access more muted and suppressed narratives in their lives. Some of the principles of narrative therapy have been applied in a wide range of settings, including family medical practice (Shapiro, 2002; Freeman & Couchonnal, 2006).

Narrative therapy makes a number of assumptions about people and problems that help practitioners to enact their roles in non-traditional ways. These include the following:

- People are experts in their own stories, which means that practitioners take a non-expert stance and try to elicit meanings rather than problems, diagnoses or labels. This approach entails respect for the stories of the people you support. In direct work, this may mean taking time to listen and ask questions about the unfolding stories of service users. When you have only indirect or cursory contact with people, it is important to bear in mind that through your interaction with them, you are becoming part of their stories. How would you like to influence their life-narratives?

- In narrative approaches, people are encouraged to name their own stories and to externalise their problems. Their problems are viewed as stories they have agreed to tell themselves and those in the business of helping them. Part of the practitioner's role is simply to listen to these narratives and acknowledge them as legitimate experiences that have meaning to the person involved. In addition, narrative practice entails using service users' own language in referring to their problems rather than professional language. Since problems are externalised and encapsulated in stories, the basic motto of narrative practice is: 'People are not the problem, the problem is the problem' (Sween, 1998).

- Service users are encouraged to explore their own stories. This means that narrative practitioners are eager to find out how elements of the story interact. Stories are explored with curiosity, and questions such as 'What would be different if…?' yield valuable insights into how people author their lives. Sometimes the stories of those needing help are characterised by overriding or dominant discourses that powerfully shape their actions or the possibilities they see open to themselves. These can be social or societal discourses (racism, for example), the narrative imposed by a domineering or abusive partner, or a strongly held personal belief ('I am a failure'; 'I am stupid'). Encouraging people to explore these narratives and their power over them is an important step in helping people break free from these oppressive narratives. In this regard, it might be helpful to think about what outcomes are prevalent in the stories of those you work with. Are the stories you routinely hear ones of failure and despair, or of success and resilience?

- Narrative practitioners work with people to re-author their lives, often focusing on exceptions to the problem. Very few people have always failed at everything they attempted. Starting with the stories about exceptions to the rule can be one way to start helping someone see different possibilities that might be open to them. Some examples include exploring situations in which people felt competent or strong rather than inadequate and weak; and past experiences of coping well and resolving dilemmas effectively rather than failures and defeats. This enables individuals to reconnect to their strengths and activate their internal resources.

- Narrative practitioners make extensive use of exploratory questions and remain curious about how service users construct their lives and the meanings that events and relationships have for them. This is in contrast to many traditional expert roles where people are told what is wrong with them (diagnosis) and then have treatments applied to them.

REFLECTIVE ACTIVITY

1. Review each of the points above and reflect on how you can apply them in your role. How would your practice be different if you worked in this way?

2. The work you do in supervision comprises your unfolding story about the people you work with. How do you represent their narratives in supervision? Would the conversation with your supervisor be different if you externalised and named their problems in the way narrative approaches suggest, in contrast to traditional views of people as the problem? From what you have learned in this chapter, are there ways in which you can use supervision differently to help people you work with more effectively to re-author their lives?

3. What is the impact of your own storymaking on your work? This includes your own story as an individual, as well as the narratives you construct about your service and its partner agencies. Think, for instance, of the ways in which many professionals construct the stories of partner agencies in negative ways.

FOR THE JOURNAL

Create and write down an illustrated story for your service and your role within it.

CHAPTER SUMMARY

Five key points to take away from Chapter 3:

- People are inherently storytellers. The rich traditions of folk tales, myths and oral histories from around the world illustrate this. When service users tell their stories, they are constructing the narratives through which they want practitioners to understand their lives and their needs.

- Many aspects of frontline practice can be constructed as narratives; for instance, the stories told about service users on referral forms and at meetings, the stories told in assessments, reports and in supervision. By virtue of these stories that practitioners tell, they have great power in co-constructing people's lives.

- By remaining aware of people's stories and the stories of their involvement with services, practitioners can show sensitivity to the impact of societal narratives on people's lives (for instance, marginalisation, discrimination and exclusion). The way in which practitioners interact with service users' narratives through their work, can promote or inhibit competence and self-esteem in service users.

↪ Organisations also have stories about the people who use their services and about each other. This can lead to opportunities for co-constructing positive narratives, but it can also lead to practitioners getting caught up in stories of scapegoating and blame.

↪ Narrative approaches within psychotherapy provide useful ideas for practitioners about how they can work with service users to construct positive outcomes for themselves through showing respect for people's stories. Practitioners can allow service users to tell their own stories in their own language and to find narratives of resilience in their stories that might enable them to move beyond present realities to a better future.

FURTHER READING

If you would like to explore narrative approaches further, there are many good and easily accessible resources available. A good place to start is to read the short paper by Sween (1998). The narrative approach to working with families, children and adolescents has been popularised by Michael White, an Australian family therapist. His books are excellent sources of practical information on using this approach and are widely available. *Maps of Narrative Practice* (White, 2007) would be an excellent way to follow up the material covered in this chapter.

04

SHAPING PEOPLE'S LIVES PART ONE: ATTACHMENT AND FAMILY INFLUENCES

CHAPTER AIMS:

In this chapter, we start to focus on family influences that shape us. We start by taking a closer look at the dynamics of the interactions between caregivers and children during early life. The topics covered are:

- The origins of attachment behaviour;

- Parental responsiveness and attachment behaviour;

- Internal working models and their impact on early and subsequent relationships;

- Infant attachment styles and their manifestations in adults;

- Attachment styles and service users.

Understanding the forces that shape people's lives and incorporating that awareness into the way you construe your encounters at work is a key aspect of your development as a reflective practitioner. This chapter and *Chapter 5* aim to help you get started on a journey towards understanding better the many ways in which individuals' motivation, personalities, and responses might be affected by factors outside their immediate control or awareness. Reflective practitioners continually strive to understand better the people they serve, while at the same time developing the ability to locate themselves and their own internal dynamics within their frames of understanding. In this chapter you will be asked to consider both of these factors: how their attachment histories may have influenced service users and their responses to services, on the one hand, and on the other, how your attachment history might affect your approach to your work.

INFANT ATTACHMENT: WHERE DOES IT ALL START?

A baby born of a desired pregnancy is likely to be welcome in the world and carry a largely positive meaning for caregivers. Unwanted or inconvenient pregnancies, on the other hand, may cause expectant mothers (and fathers) much distress. It is also unlikely that a child who is born into an emotionally fraught environment will be able to escape the impact of the distress that surrounds him or her. However, the story of infant attachment starts even earlier than pregnancy.

Parents' fantasies, wishes, and dreams for themselves and their lives feed into the way in which an expectant woman relates to the developing foetus. Family narratives about the unborn child start to be constructed when or even before the pregnancy becomes known within the wider family. For many, if not all infants, there is already in existence, by the time they are born, a whole web of meaning that surrounds their arrival into the world. An important part of this web of meaning is the meaning the infant has for its caregivers. And it stands to reason that the caregivers' images of their infant shape their reaction to and responsiveness in relation to their child.

The story of attachment starts with this web of meaning that surrounds the newborn baby. Depending on the way in which the infant's existence and behaviour is constructed in the minds of its carers, unconditional acceptance may follow, or the infant might experience the conditions under which nurturing attention is available. Adherents of attachment theory believe that the resulting relationship patterns form the prototypes for subsequent patterns of relating and provide a template for the conditions under which the individual will feel valued, loved and accepted.

REFLECTIVE ACTIVITY

Think of examples from your own experience – in your extended family, with acquaintances, or from work – of the kinds of expectations that develop in families about children, even before birth. Taking your cue from *Chapters 2* and *3*, what are the influences of family structure, history and family narratives on these? How can such expectations affect the emotional development of children? How can awareness of these influences in people you work with, enhance your practice?

THE KEY TO SECURITY: PARENTAL RESPONSIVENESS

Through their experience of their parents' responses to them, babies and young children soon develop a sense of their own value and their place in the world. They may find that their needs are met with joy and that they receive unconditional love and warmth. Alternatively, parental responses may reflect 'rules' such as 'I love you only when you are no trouble', 'Children should be seen and not heard', or 'You're in the way'. When a baby's needs are met, but with parental resentment, the message may be 'Don't exist', or one of blame: 'It's your fault that I'm stuck at home, unable to live my life'.

Attachment theory is a theory of human development and personality which takes as a starting point the notion that our earliest experiences in relationships can have a very powerful impact on our subsequent psychological functioning. Infants are completely dependent on their caregivers for their basic needs. One of nature's ways of equipping newborn babies for survival is to 'hard wire' them with a repertoire of behaviours designed to elicit caring and contact from their caregivers. Crying and cooing are examples of these attachment behaviours because babies use these behaviours to elicit caring, soothing or social responses from their caregivers. Part of the reason why attachment behaviour and the consequent caregiver responses are such powerful shaping influences on human relationship behaviour is because attachment behaviour is generated by survival needs. For an infant, being taken care of and having fundamental needs of shelter, warmth, protection and nourishment met is, quite literally, a matter of life and death!

Caregivers respond in different ways to these signals that infants send. Studies of attachment behaviour and the accompanying caregiver responses in infants have highlighted the following four dimensions of parental responsiveness (Howe, Brandon, Hinings & Schofield, 1999). Parents can respond differently to their children at different times and under different circumstances, so where someone falls on these dimensions is a dynamic and changeable profile:

- **Sensitivity–insensitivity:** Caregivers who are sensitive to the needs of their infants react to the child's signals, while parents towards the insensitive end of the continuum tend not to acknowledge or be aware of the signals their baby is sending. The messages from consistently sensitive parental responses to infants are that 'You are important' and 'Your needs count'.

- **Acceptance–rejection:** This dimension is about caregiver acknowledgement that the child's needs are legitimate. The message to the infant is one which accepts the infant's own expression of his or her bodily signals by responding to the subsequent attachment behaviour. Accepting parental responses indicates to infants that their request for proximity, contact or comfort is viewed as legitimate and responded to in a way that meets their underlying needs. With acceptance of the baby's needs for care comes parental validation of their infants' existence.

  At the opposite end of the continuum, the messages to a child from a caregiver who responds to attachment behaviour in a rejecting style could be 'I wish you weren't here' or 'Only I know what you need; you don't'.

- **Cooperation–interference**: This dimension refers to the extent to which caregivers facilitate the meeting of their infants' needs, especially relating to their emerging attempts to develop independence skills. Caregivers who respond cooperatively reinforce infants' attempts at practising emerging skills. Cooperative caregivers are accepting of children's first, faltering attempts at mastery. They reinforce trying, even if the child is not successful for a while. The child develops a sense of agency, i.e. 'I can make a difference to my world' and of mastery; 'I can'.

Caregivers who consistently undermine or interfere with their children's attempts at self-sufficiency create in their children a sense of uncertainty and self-doubt. These children may explore less and respond with dependency, give up or despair when they struggle to solve problems they encounter. They may end up mistrustful of their own emotions and abilities. Interference in this sense can also come from well-meaning parents who may, for instance, curb a toddler's exploring behaviour, due to their fear of the dangers that the child might encounter.

- **Accessible–ignoring:** This dimension relates to how available caregivers are to their children. Caregivers who are consistently accessible and available foster in their children a sense of security and safety. Children whose caregivers are consistently unavailable, or only inconsistently available, may find it difficult to make sense of exactly what it would take to gain caring responses to their attachment behaviour. This may lead them to develop response patterns that maximise their chances of eliciting a response, or, if caregivers are consistently unresponsive, they may give up trying.

REFLECTIVE ACTIVITY

How might the following issues in caregivers' lives affect their ability to respond to their infants' attachment behaviours?

a) Post-natal depression

b) Substance abuse

c) Domestic violence

In your answer, try to take account of the different dimensions mentioned above. What might the resultant messages of these parental response styles be from the child's perspective? To get you started: a mother who is subject to domestic violence may only be inconsistently available to her infant, due to periods of fear for her own safety and the incidents of violence she is subject to. From the child's perspective this may lead to periods when crying is ignored or responded to with fear, alternating with periods when needs are met with sensitivity and acceptance.

DEVELOPING A SENSE OF SELF: THE INTERNAL WORKING MODEL

Through experiencing their parents' responses to them, infants soon acquire a sense of whether they are accepted unconditionally, only under certain circumstances, or not at all.

They learn what they have to do in order to get their caregivers to take notice of them, and whether or not the world around them is a safe and happy place, or dangerous, or unpredictable and inconsistent.

These expectations develop into a set of mental representations that attachment theorists refer to as internal working models (Ainsworth, Blehar, Waters & Wall, 1978). An internal working model consists of a set of expectations about self, about others and about the world.

Self: Expectations about the self determine infants' emerging sense of identity, their capabilities, and their physical and psychological boundaries.

Others: The expectations we develop about others include a general sense of whether people are safe and trustworthy, how they behave towards us, what we need to do to please them, and how to get them to take notice of us.

The world: The third component of the internal working model is a general sense of what we can expect from the world around us. Is the world a safe place or is it dangerous? Do good things generally happen to me, or is the world full of frightening events?

In infancy, this element of the internal working model is especially affected by caregivers' responses to young children's early attempts at exploration. If these are encouraged and praised, children are likely to develop a sense of security about the 'self in the world'. If not, children are likely to sense their caregivers' apprehension or anxiety and inhibit their exploratory behaviour in response.

Where children feel encouraged to explore and to try out new behaviours, caregivers have created in the child a sense of themselves as an anchor point, a secure base from which their infants can explore safely.

Internal working models as blueprints for relationships

Over time these internal working models become self-perpetuating. We act in ways that elicit the expected and usual responses from others which, in turn, lead to 'the usual' feelings and responses from us. This, in turn, can influence the behaviour of others towards us, thus perpetuating the process. If you have ever been in a situation where you, a service user or an acquaintance exclaimed 'Why does this always happen to me?' you are probably seeing an internal working model in action (Howe, Brandon, Hinings & Schofield, 1999).

Our internal working models generally operate outside the realm of conscious awareness. Clues as to what constitute our general expectations regarding self, others and the world can be found through identifying recurring patterns of behaviour or outcomes in our lives, rules for living and those sayings our parents or grandparents may have repeated so frequently that they have become ingrained in our consciousness. For example, you may find that you are always disappointed in the trustworthiness of friends. Rules for living can include 'Be perfect', 'Other people will only accept me if I please them', or 'Don't trust anyone'. Sayings that may arise in families could be, for example, 'It is not worth doing if it is not done well', or 'Children should be seen and not heard'. In *Chapter 5*, we look at some of the factors in a family's history that might shape these messages and slogans.

As we shall see in the following two reflective activities, internal working models can be very powerful influences both on practitioners' own dynamics within the workplace, and the ways in which service users respond to services. Reflective practitioners work from within an awareness of the ways in which their own inner theatres affect their practice. They also remain mindful of how aspects of service users' psychological dynamics can affect their responses to services. An interesting feature of the ways in which internal working models can affect these two very disparate factors (i.e. practitioners' relationship patterns in the workplace, and service users' responses to services) is that, in both cases, where a response originates in an individual's internal working model, that response is likely to represent a relationship pattern that is displaced from an earlier relationship into the present. As such these displaced responses are not necessarily rational responses to the situations at hand and they can leave recipients feeling confused or puzzled as to the cause of the reaction. The second reflective activity below serves to illustrate this point a little further. In *Chapter 10*, we explore the impact of displaced emotions in greater depth when we consider transference and countertransference reactions.

REFLECTIVE ACTIVITY

Can you think of relationship patterns, rules for living or family slogans that have become a part of how you view the world? How have these affected the way in which you live your life? The answers to these questions will help you make a start at finding out more about what is contained in your own internal working model. It might also be fruitful to explore your internal working model specifically with regard to how it impacts on work. To get you started, you might wish to consider the following questions:

- Which self-expectations influence your behaviour at work? These could be things such as the need to complete even mundane tasks perfectly, or a tendency to expect failure when placed under pressure.

- What do you expect from others in the work context and does what you routinely get back in return match your expectations?

- What is your pattern of relating to authority figures? Can you relate that back to people in your past, e.g. parents, teachers, and so on?

- Are there areas of your work life where you feel you experience a repeated pattern? Can you think of how your internal working model may contribute to that?

This activity is continued in the journalling exercise for this chapter.

REFLECTIVE ACTIVITY

All of the people who use your services have their own internal working models. The main point of this chapter is that their expectations regarding self, others and the world will affect how they respond to you and your service.

Consider the following vignette:

Josie is 25 and a single mum. She has recently been referred to a family support team at a local Children's Centre after she told the teacher at her daughter's nursery that she struggles to get her child to bed at night. Below are three possible examples of how Josie's internal working model might lead her to view herself, others and the world.

Table 4.1 *Josie's internal working model: three possible scenarios*

Internal working model:	Scenario A	Scenario B	Scenario C
Self	I am OK	I am OK	I am not OK. I am not very successful in life
Others	People are generally helpful and accepting.	People generally cannot be trusted – everyone has an agenda.	Other people are generally helpful; Others are generally more competent than me.
The world	Things usually work out for me.	Things would work out for me, if others only would stop meddling.	The world is a bit of a daunting place; I am fortunate I made it through life so far because everything is very confusing.

I. For each of these three scenarios, answer the following questions:

1. How might Josie feel about her referral for services? How is she likely to respond to the practitioner allocated to her? What would be her most likely view of the offer of support?

2. If she is reluctant to engage with the service, how would you deal with that in each of the above scenarios?

3. How is Josie likely to respond to advice given? What might she do if things did not get better straight away?

4. How is she likely to respond to the work ending in each of these scenarios? How would you manage your work with her ending in each case?

II. Make a list of some questions to ask, or observations you could make, that might help you determine early on in your involvement with someone what their internal working model might be as it relates to you, your service, and the difficulty at hand.

III. Look back at scenarios B and C regarding Josie. Which of these would be easiest for you to work with and which would be the most difficult? Why? Is there something in your own internal working model that is triggered by certain responses of service users? How can you use that knowledge to develop your own professional practice?

ATTACHMENT STYLES: PATTERNS OF RELATING THAT STICK

Experimental studies by Mary Ainsworth and her co-workers (Ainsworth, Blehar, Waters & Wall, 1978) uncovered a number of broad attachment styles. Most individuals can be classified as falling into one of these patterns. Attachment styles represent the habitual or organised ways in which an individual has learned he or she should behave in order to get their basic needs met. For infants this may include such learning as 'Crying only helps sometimes', or 'In order to be heard, I have to kick up a huge fuss'. Over time, as the same behaviours elicit predictable caregiver responses, stable patterns develop. As infants grow older, the patterns may persist, although the behaviour that constitutes them may become more sophisticated. For example, a baby who learns that only loud, persistent crying gets any response may subsequently develop an emotionally dramatic style of behaving. A baby who learns that crying does not really help may suppress expressions of distress. In the long run this might lead to denying or suppressing strong emotions, responding instead to distress with rationalisation.

Although the original research was done with young children, subsequent studies have expanded the age range for which these attachment patterns are valid. Attachment theorists believe that adults use these attachment styles within the close relationships they develop with others. As such, individual attachment styles may also affect the ways in which people respond to frontline services, especially if the meeting of fundamental human survival needs is at stake. The definition of frontline services as applied throughout this book was given in the Introduction as exactly this: services that deal with vulnerable people's needs for safety and shelter, and physical, mental and psychological health.)

The descriptions that follow provide an outline of the major identified attachment styles, following Ainsworth's research. This is not the only or most comprehensive way to classify attachment styles, but it has stood the test of time. Each style is briefly described as it applies to infants or children in the original observations, and then some implications are drawn regarding how someone with this attachment style might respond to services.

Secure attachment style

Original observations: Securely attached children are free to explore and play as they perceive their caregivers as a secure base. Distress is effectively dealt with by caregivers who are able to soothe and calm the child quickly, while there is an appropriate level of apprehension regarding strangers.

Presentation to services: Individuals with secure attachment styles are likely to be able to relate effectively to services and practitioners. They show a balanced ability to express emotion and rational thought and can therefore 'use' practitioners effectively. They are able to balance distress with the expectation that intervention will help, and they appreciate the need for endings and moving on to being more self-sufficient.

Insecure–avoidant attachment style

Original observations: Children are relatively self-contained with limited attachment behaviour expressed. It is as if signals were muted because they were being ignored by caregivers. In later childhood this might lead to over-rationalisation and being out of touch with emotions or unable to express distress. These children may feel anxious in the presence of strong emotions and tend not to rely on others for feeling secure.

Presentation to services: These individuals are likely to deny the impact of difficulties on them and underrate the extent to which they need help. They are guarded and avoid feeling strong emotions. They are also reluctant to ask for help or report difficulties that occur along the way. Thoughts and emotions are often separated, creating a sense that thinking is used to cover up feelings.

Insecure–ambivalent attachment style

Original observations: Infants who learned that caregivers were likely to respond only if needs were expressed intensively and for prolonged periods of time are likely to fall into this category. There is often an interpersonal ambivalence present. In the early attachment research which included episodes of separation from a caregiver, many infants in this group responded with reduced exploration of their environments and anger/tantrums directed at caregivers on being reunited. The prevailing pattern is one of alternately feeling love and anger for attachment figures combined with a very dramatic presentation. It seems that ambivalent attachment predisposes individuals to present in emotionally dramatic and impulsive ways, where thinking is inhibited in favour of feeling.

Presentation to services: Individuals may present in dramatic ways with high levels of expressed emotion. Rational problem solving may be a particular challenge, as would be maintaining stable dependency relationships with others. Anger at perceived past rejections may affect engagement with services. These individuals feel very insecure about their own lovability and value. They find it very difficult to use rational thinking to help them manage their strong emotions. They may also use coercive strategies and life crises to get a response from services.

Disorganised attachment styles

Original observations: These attachment styles could originally not be classified, as the children concerned had not shown a consistent strategy to gain caregiver responses. Subsequently, this category has been used to describe individuals whose early attachment histories have been so chaotic that no consistent strategy worked for them. They may therefore use a range of ways in which to elicit nurturing and care, including role reversal ('parentification' of the child) and coercive, punitive, compulsively compliant, disinhibited or inhibited presentations (Howe, Brandon, Hinings & Schofield, 1999).

Presentation to services: These individuals may present as chaotic, difficult clients. Their responses to practitioners may be unpredictable and varied. They may attempt to manipulate the service provider–service recipient relationship in ways consistent with their personal relationship history; for example, by compulsive compliance, attempting to take care of the practitioner, or even complete non-engagement. For practitioners, there may be a very substantial discrepancy between the response they would ordinarily expect from individuals with similar needs and the particular service recipient's response to their efforts.

REFLECTIVE ACTIVITY

1. Go through the list of people you currently work with. Are there any who, to your mind, clearly fall into one of these attachment style categories? What makes you think that? What do you know about their personal histories that confirms your hunch? What is the contrary evidence?

2. How can understanding someone's attachment style help you be more effective in your work role? For example, would knowing that someone is prone to minimising the emotional impact of their difficulties – insecure–avoidant style – impact on your approach? How would you work differently with someone who regularly presents in the dramatic way described earlier for people with an ambivalent attachment style?

3. What about people who fall in the disorganised attachment style category? How would you work differently with someone who, for instance, wants to keep taking care of you? An example of this might be through showing excessive concern for your wellbeing or excessive gift giving.

There are three aspects of the work in frontline services where you are most likely to see the impact of service users' attachment styles. The first is in the ways that individuals express distress. As mentioned above, while individuals who exhibit a secure attachment style are able to balance thought and emotion in the way they process information, individuals with attachment difficulties may find this very hard. People with avoidant styles may suppress strong feelings and may be very reluctant to admit that they are finding it difficult to cope. Service users with ambivalent styles may present as over-dramatic, and problem solving with them may be very difficult. Feelings of being overwhelmed may be hard to shift, even if rational solutions to difficulties are readily available. Setbacks along the way may feel overwhelming and these individuals may feel that it would be impossible to solve their problems. Catastrophic reactions may include outbursts of anger at practitioners for not succeeding in sorting out their problems for them.

In individuals with disorganised, coercive styles, the predominant attitude may be that solving the issues behind their referral to your service, is entirely your problem. Compulsively compliant individuals may accept professionals' definitions of their difficulties without question, but practitioners may feel quite unsure about the extent to which their concerns are genuinely shared or accepted as valid by the person concerned, as their compliance appears to have an exaggerated and superficial quality to it.

The second area of frontline practice in which attachment style is likely to play a role is that of maintaining key relationships. Unattached (disorganised–inhibited) individuals and those with avoidant styles are unlikely to make good use of relationships with practitioners or therapists to help them change. Their attachment histories have taught them that their needs are not routinely met within relationships and that therefore they only have themselves to rely on. This may imply that practitioners should focus on problem solving approaches for short-term work, while medium- to long-term psychotherapy may be the only way to address core issues regarding relating to others. In contrast, ambivalent individuals may be very dependent on their relationships with others to help them solve problems requiring rational thought, but their dramatic behaviour within dependency relationships may cause tension and relationship breakdowns. The challenge for practitioners is to support the individual to maintain their relationships with services, despite potentially dramatic conflicts with practitioners.

The third key area concerns dealing with endings. Individuals with attachment histories that involve having little experience of secure, nurturing relationships are likely to find endings very difficult (provided, of course, that they built up a good relationship with the service concerned over time.) In the chapter on boundaries (*Chapter 6*), I make the point that considering endings should be part of the work with service users right from the start of any service's involvement.

For individuals with insecurity about their value and lovability, it is important to make sure that the successful conclusion of a piece of work is not followed by acute feelings of distress at the loss of a key relationship in the service user's life. This also affects transfers of cases between team members. A service user's angry response to a new team member taking on their case may be an expression of distress at the loss of relationship with the previous practitioner. In contrast, in services that rely on service users themselves to signal the need for involvement to end, people with avoidant or inhibited attachment may terminate work prematurely. Practitioners may close these cases with a sense of unease about the adequacy of the amount of progress made.

REFLECTIVE ACTIVITY

To what extent do you agree or disagree with the perspectives presented here on how attachment styles can manifest themselves in service users' responses to services? Can you think of factors other than the ones mentioned here that can lead to service users finding it difficult to ask for help appropriately, maintain relationships, or deal with endings?

What are your views on how practitioner attachment styles affect these three key areas of practice? (Expression of distress, maintaining key relationships, dealing with endings)

A final word of caution: the information on the different attachment styles presented here does not form a comprehensive account of attachment theory. While the material in the text is presented with the aim of helping readers to understand better some of the psychological processes in themselves and service users, you should always remain open to the possibility that there might be an alternative explanation for someone's behaviour. This is especially true for any system that classifies people into categories and then draws inferences about the causes of their behaviour, based on their classification. Considering someone's attachment style as a potential explanation for their behaviour may be helpful in many cases, but it will not be perfectly accurate in all situations. Conclusions drawn from categorising people should therefore always be viewed as very tentative and subject to confirmation with evidence from real life.

FOR THE JOURNAL

Continue with the activity that you started earlier in the chapter on your own internal working model.

Over the next few weeks, try to note down in your journal anything you learn about the way your own internal working model operates. It might be especially helpful to focus on factors relating to work. It might also be helpful to note when your interactions with colleagues or service users lead you to experience unexpectedly strong feelings or outcomes that, on reflection, appear to be consistent with a repeating pattern. These may be clues that your internal working model is operating.

Once you have noted some of your work-related expectations regarding self, others and the world, reflect on the implications for yourself in terms of your career development. Does this raise any professional development needs for you to address over the next twelve months?

CHAPTER SUMMARY

Five key points to take away from Chapter 4:

- Effective reflective practice includes developing the ability to apply a conceptual understanding of the forces that shape service users' lives and those of practitioners. Attachment theories are helpful in informing our understanding of how early relationships shape our subsequent patterns of behaviour and our relationships with others and ourselves.

- Attachment theory provides an explanation of behaviour that draws on the power of caregiver responsiveness to infants' attachment signals (e.g. crying) to shape expectations regarding what it takes to be protected, comforted and valued. This early learning process shapes our subsequent expectations for how others and the world will respond to us and how we need to behave to have our needs met.

- Different attachment styles represent strategies that infants develop in order to deal with danger in their environments. The resulting patterns of relating can affect how individuals respond to services in areas such as establishing helping relationships with practitioners, responding to advice, and managing boundaries.

- Different attachment styles may lead to different responses to services. Possible patterns are:

  - Secure attachment style: rational and realistic

  - Insecure–avoidant: insular/independent relationship style; defends against emotions by focusing on rationalisation

  - Insecure–ambivalent: dependent and unsure of own lovability in relationships; defends against rational thinking through taking an emotion-focused approach

  - Disorganised: can present in a chaotic way, tending to get trapped in compulsive compliance, or coercive strategies in relationships and problem solving.

- Reflective practitioners also cultivate awareness of their own attachment styles and how these influence their approach to service users. When reflection on their practice indicates the need, they use supervision and support effectively to address issues and improve their practice – see *Part Four* of this book for further coverage of supervision, team support, and dealing with stress and burnout.

FURTHER READING

There is much more to attachment theory than the ground covered in this chapter. If you would like an accessible and practical introduction to attachment perspectives, Heather Geddes' book *Attachment in the Classroom* (2006) is hard to beat. The book covers the basic theory and applies it to the classroom setting, but some of the points raised are applicable across all the settings which children and families access.

For a more academic introduction from social work and child protection perspectives, the book by David Howe *et al.* referenced in the text would provide an excellent starting point. The authors present a detailed overview of attachment theory, information on how to assess attachment styles, and also discuss the implications of different attachment styles across different age groups.

05

SHAPING PEOPLE'S LIVES PART TWO: CROSS-GENERATIONAL INFLUENCES AND MIGRATION

THIS CHAPTER AIMS TO:

- Explore the impact of family history and the internal dynamics of family life on individuals' sense of their identity;

- Explore the impact of migration on identity;

- Introduce you to the impact of historical trauma and displacement on families across generations;

- Raise your awareness of how your own history interacts with those of people who use your services.

FAMILY HISTORY AND PERSONAL IDENTITY

Take a few minutes to come up with as many answers as you can think of to the following questions, 'Who am I? What is my personal identity?' What did you come up with? Most of us in Western societies are likely to think of our identity firstly in terms of our individual traits or characteristics: 'I am a social worker', 'I am confident' or 'I have little self confidence', 'I am good at my job', 'I am outgoing' or 'I am introverted', and so on. Perhaps you thought of an affiliation such as your culture, religion, or a group you belong to. However, my guess is that you thought of yourself firstly in terms of your individual traits. Yet each of us is, in part, also the product of our own and our families' histories. The contention in this chapter is that, to a surprising extent, history – your history – goes with you wherever you go, and can even have a strong influence on those behaviours or traits you may think of as individual to you. The same may be true of the people who use your services.

Following on from the introductory exercise above, what do you know about your family history, one, two or even three generations back? How did you end up in the geographical area where you grew up? Is there a story of migration or loss of home in your family, either for yourself or any of the previous generations? Or has your family stayed in the same community for generations? What do you know about the history and the impact this may have had on you or the previous generations of your family? Are there any relatives or ancestors who feature prominently in the family's account of their history and what stories are told about them?

If there is a history of migration in your family, you may find that even the second or third generation is affected. For example, children of parents who have fled very traumatic situations in their home countries may find that their parents have carried over to their new homes some of the survival strategies that served them well in their countries of origin, and these may no longer be helpful or relevant. The emotional climate in a family as well as the family narrative can be hugely affected by such cultural or historical factors.

The previous exercise asked you to reflect on your own sense of identity and your family history. It is generally accepted nowadays that where you come from can have a huge impact on many aspects of your life, from your chances of surviving infancy and childhood through to your eventual prospects for economic advancement as an adult. Without the benefit of state intervention, the socio-economic status of your parents will strongly affect the educational opportunities and life experiences available to you. The same goes for your life chances if your ethnic or cultural group is part of the accepted groups in the mainstream of your society, or discriminated against or marginalised (UNICEF, 2009).

Within a cultural milieu where gender roles are sharply defined and rigidly enforced, whether you are male or female can determine the opportunities available to you, and your eventual life course. Within a family context, whether you are an only child or one of many children may also have a huge impact on your childhood experiences and opportunities. The place where many of these forces enact their influence on individuals' destinies is family life, and the family can therefore be viewed as an institution that socialises individuals into accepted social roles.

In the rest of this chapter, we will consider a number of ideas that help us to come to an understanding of how family history impacts on people across generations. In the next section, we will consider the fundamental family tasks that underlie the functioning of all families. The section that follows examines the migration process, followed by a focus on the intergenerational transmission of traumatic experiences and the impact these can have on individuals. The closing section focuses on the interaction between the histories of service users and practitioners.

UNDERSTANDING FAMILY DYNAMICS: FOUR CENTRAL FAMILY TASKS

REFLECTIVE ACTIVITY

Imagine your family having a meal together. Who is present? How do people occupy the physical space within which you are gathered? For example, who sits where at the table? Do specific family members have special tasks or roles? Who talks and about what, who listens, and who dissents? What do the communication patterns around the table tell you about the way your family works? If you are attempting this exercise in a group, everyone can make a drawing or a diagram that shows this scene in their family to share with the group. Which elements of how things worked in your family are illustrated by your drawing or account of your family at a meal?

When the family is viewed as an institution, research has shown that family dynamics are shaped by the ways in which a family resolves the following four challenges (Hess & Handel, 1967).

Developing a congruent set of images

Family members form internal 'emotional' images of each other and of themselves. These images reflect how each person views him or herself in relation to the other family members and their perceptions of their interactions with one another within the family context. This can include labelling within the family as well as perceptions related to illness, disability, or favouritism. For a family to function effectively, there needs to be a certain degree of congruence between different members' imagery of one another. For example, many families would respond very differently to the difficult behaviour of children perceived to be on the autism spectrum, compared to children viewed as being difficult or defiant.

Evolving a central family theme and relevant modes of family interaction

Related to their internal set of images of one another, families also develop a definition of themselves *as a family* in relation to the external world. The family 'theme' involves those unspoken rules or standards of conduct that family members apply to one another within the family. Family themes can relate to religion or culture as well as to the family's account of their history. Family themes can also relate to behaviour that is allowed or disallowed between family members; for example, who is allowed to disagree with whom in the family, or who is consulted when decisions are made.

Establishing boundaries around the family's world of experience

This task relates to the permeability of family boundaries towards the outside world. Which influences are allowed in and which are barred? Who is free to leave and who has to stay? What happens to you if you choose to leave the family home?

Dealing with significant developmental and biological issues in the family's life

All families go through a life cycle that is linked to the biology of family members. How does the family make sense of and deal with pregnancy, infants and young children, teenagers, getting older, and sickness or disability in individual family members?

Successfully completing these tasks at different stages of the family life cycle allows functioning families and their members to form a coherent sense of family identity. When families are dysfunctional, it is often possible to understand their difficulties better by referring to these tasks and considering the ways in which they have constructed their mutual images, family theme, relationship to the outside world, and how they managed the developmental/biological challenges they faced in life.

REFLECTIVE ACTIVITY

Think of an example of a family you have worked with and try to describe your observations of them in terms of the above categories: family members' images of one another, the central family theme and interactions, boundaries with the external world, and developmental or biological issues in the family's life. If the family was dysfunctional in some way, could you encapsulate their difficulties under these headings? What about describing their strengths?

REFLECTIVE ACTIVITY

Are there commonalities across these four areas in the families you work with? Would taking time to think about family dynamics using the four family tasks described here help you in your service?

MOVING AWAY, MAKING A NEW LIFE: THE EXPERIENCE OF MIGRATION

As mentioned earlier in this chapter, migration, the process of making a new home somewhere geographically distant from one's place of origin, is an increasingly common experience in the background of service users and practitioners alike. For some families, migration consists of moving half-way across the world and adapting to a completely new cultural and social milieu. For other families, the very same process of adjusting to a change in environment and culture can take place when they move from one county to the next, or even between different parts of the same city.

Migration in all its forms can be an unsettling and stressful experience. Research into the psychology and impact of migration on migrants has highlighted a number of challenges that people encounter at different stages of the process (Bhugra & Jones, 2001). Prior to migration, the challenges involve preparation and planning for migration. Stress can arise from a variety of factors including the reason for leaving, challenges in the preparation process, difficulties with obtaining the relevant documentation, and the impact of saying goodbye to friends, family and other sources of social support.

During the journey, some migrants face danger and risk. In other cases people are alone and acutely aware of the uncertainties they face upon arrival at their final destination.

Post-migration, there is a process of assimilation in the new environment and acculturation; the process of getting used to a new society, different ways of doing things, and local culture, can be very stressful, even for individuals who move to different areas within their countries of origin. Over time, migrants also tend to give up or lose some aspects of their original cultures. This process of deculturation can leave people feeling that they belong neither to the society they originally came from nor to their host culture. This phenomenon has been described as 'cultural bereavement' (Eisenbruch, 1991).

For people who have migrated over very long distances or between countries where the host cultures are very different from the cultures in the migrants' countries of origin, cultural bereavement can be a very significant factor in the wellbeing of migrants. So, for instance, refugees from Asian countries finding asylum in western Europe or the USA can report 'symptoms' that sound very bizarre to practitioners who are not culturally aware. For example, Eisenbruch (1991) found among Cambodian refugees that cultural bereavement can lead to people 'living in the past' and feeling guilty about leaving their homes. Positive memories from the past can fade, and migrants can feel a sense of wanting to fulfil their obligations to their relatives in their countries of origin, whether living or dead, and experience supernatural visitations from their ancestors. Some of these symptoms can be mistaken for psychiatric illness, but Western medical approaches are not generally helpful. Instead, supporting people to access appropriate religious and cultural ceremonies appears to be the approach of choice in these situations.

REFLECTIVE ACTIVITY

Try to think of someone you know who has experienced migration or relocation that involved going through the three-stage process described above. How would you characterise the challenges they faced pre-migration, during the migration process, and afterwards? Do you think any of these stressors affected them severely enough for them to need services?

What about yourself? The same process applies to anyone who moves elsewhere to start a new life. Have you gone through a process where you had to leave loved ones behind to go and live somewhere else? What was that like? You can use the above framework to reflect on your life experiences. If you haven't had a migration experience, perhaps you might like to think about what you anticipate may be the challenges you would face if you were to become a migrant.

How might the migration experience affect the way someone presents to your service? Can you think of an incident you can do a CLT cycle for?

FAMILY IDENTITY, MIGRATION AND HISTORICAL TRAUMA: CAN TRAUMA BE TRANSMITTED ACROSS GENERATIONS?

In a culturally diverse society such as ours, migration is a common occurrence and staff in frontline services often come into contact with service users whose history includes movement across international borders. People migrate for a large variety of reasons, including escape from traumatic situations such as genocide and ethnic or religious persecution. Apart from the direct effects of trauma on the individuals concerned, there might also be an indirect, cross-generational effect on children of the second and even the third generations.

The idea that trauma can be transmitted across generations was first mooted when case studies of psychotherapy with children of Holocaust survivors started to appear in the scientific literature in the 1960s. In the ensuing decades further studies were done with mixed results, some showing definite trauma in second and third generation Holocaust survivors and some research showing no evidence of this. In all, there have been over 400 studies published in the scientific literature. Reviewing this research, Kellerman (2001) concluded that, in general, the findings pointed to a specific kind of psychological profile found in the children of survivors that affected the way they coped with stress, thus making them vulnerable. More recent research has indicated that some of the findings relating to the children of Holocaust survivors also apply to people who survived other historical traumas (Kellerman, 2001).

REFLECTIVE ACTIVITY

Some of the research in this area examined the interaction patterns and caretaking within families of survivors. The following fictionalised description is based on such research (Brown, 1998; Kellerman, 2001).

'Mum and dad never told us what happened to them during the war. We only found out after dad's death that they were both in the camps. Maybe that explains their long silences and the knowing glances they shared. As children, we always found them to be stifling – they never let us have friends around for sleepovers and were always suspicious of the neighbours for no reason we could see. They only socialised with people from the old country who they knew from before. No one ever cried. We always just got on with things. There was no sympathy for the disappointments of life that afflict any child. Not getting a part in the school play or breaking up with your best friend seemed to pale into insignificance to just surviving. Nothing was ever said in our house, but we sensed it. At the same time, we always felt that we were different, not quite good enough, especially where school grades were concerned. After dad's death we found out that he studied engineering at a prestigious university before the war, but over here he worked as a shift supervisor in a tractor factory. He never complained about anything. Mum was the same, never a tear, but also very little by way of comforting words. We always felt they were somehow ashamed of us.'

Questions

1. Consider the above description of life in the home of Holocaust survivors in the light of some of the family tasks mentioned in the previous section. What might the set of family images created within this family be? What were the themes of family interaction prevalent within this family? How did the parents set the boundaries between the family and the world around them? How might the children who were not told of their parents' experiences explain the parents' behaviour to themselves? How might that affect their views of self, others, and the world in general? From this information, what are your thoughts on the likely impact of the parents' trauma on their children?

2. The last few decades have seen many historical traumas and some of the survivors of these tragedies have settled in the UK. Can you name some of these events? Have you worked with anyone who has been affected? If so, what, in your experience, was the impact on the direct victims and on their offspring?

WHEN PATHS CROSS: HOW THE HISTORIES OF SERVICE USERS INTERACT WITH THOSE OF PRACTITIONERS

The people who use your service all come from families, each with a unique family history and their own solutions to the challenges of developing congruent images, a coherent family theme, boundaries to the outside world and a response to developmental and biological challenges faced by family members. An awareness of how these factors have contributed to shaping individual family members' identities can help you hugely in building rapport, delivering effective interventions, and understanding their attitude and behaviour towards your service.

If your role allows you to talk to people about their family histories, it may be very enlightening to go back at least one generation and try to find out how the family historically dealt with the four family tasks mentioned above. Understanding the roles and choices made in each generation of a family may give you clues to the different relationship patterns available to family members and how families relate to the world around them. Awareness of repeating patterns across generations is often the first step to change, or, at the very least, an important clue to reasons why interventions may have failed in the past.

Frontline staff members who do not routinely get the opportunity to talk to families about their histories can still detect the traces of some of these patterns through careful observation and judicious questioning. In particular, carefully observing which behaviours are rewarded with validation and who has the right to voice their views may provide powerful clues to family power structures and families' themes and images as these relate to the different family members, while the responses of family members to outside agencies may be indicative of how families typically deal with boundary issues.

The final important factor to consider in this exploration of the impact of family history and dynamics on frontline practitioners is the interaction between service users' family patterns and those of practitioners. Consider the following two examples:

REFLECTIVE ACTIVITY

Amy is a newly qualified social worker in a child protection team. She is the elder of two children in a two-parent family where her mother was an alcoholic. Amy spent much of her childhood taking care of her younger sibling, preparing meals and housework to cover for her mother, and helping her mum when she was drunk. Her father worked long hours, using work as a way to avoid facing his family. Although there was always more than enough money in the home for nice things and Amy wanted for nothing material, she grew up resenting both of her parents, but for different reasons. Yet her keen sense of responsibility stopped her showing this outwardly.

She was recently sent to do an initial home visit with a young mother who was the victim of domestic abuse by a partner who was also a drug user. Her supervisor was surprised to sense a vehemence in her attitude towards the mother and was very taken aback by the strength of her conviction that the baby needed to be removed into a more caring, safe environment with responsible foster carers. Amy felt strongly about this, even though it was early in the assessment and Amy did not (yet) have any objective evidence to support her view.

John's paternal and maternal grandparents emigrated to the UK from eastern Europe over 50 years ago. Both his parents grew up in homes where their parents spoke with heavy accents and they felt unwelcome in the UK. They were not allowed to socialise with local children outside school and were only allowed to court other young people from their own culture. Although John's parents spoke English fluently and were integrated in the local community, family stories about their heritage and country of origin, as well as the obstacles to family members fitting into society in the UK, permeated his childhood. During his time at university John took part in several human rights protests. He chose to become a teacher in an inner city school with a catchment area that included many immigrant communities.

Consider the two vignettes above and answer the following questions:

1. Which aspects of their histories led/drove Amy and John to choose helping professions? How did their backgrounds affect their attitudes to their work and the groups who were their clients?

2. In what situations would Amy's need to take care of others and keen sense of responsibility be most likely to become an obstacle to her professional practice? Could John's keen awareness of people not fitting in and his sense of social justice ever get in the way of his professionalism and how would you advise him to deal with the issues that might arise?

FOR THE JOURNAL

In this chapter you were asked to do a number of exercises that challenged you to explore your own background and history. Draw all of these together in your journal by summarising your learning about the impact of your own family history and the dynamics of your family of origin on your career choice and your values as a practitioner. Are there client groups you feel particularly drawn to because of your history? Which client groups would present particular challenges to you on account of your background? How will you address those?

CHAPTER SUMMARY

Five key points to take away from Chapter 5:

- There are many factors that shape our personal identities. One set of factors that is often ignored in work with vulnerable people is the influence of family history, migration and the cross-generational transmission of trauma.

- These factors impact on family functioning through the way they influence the approach families take to accomplish the four fundamental family tasks, which are: family members forming a congruent set of images of each other, a central family theme or narrative of who they are in relation to the outside world, establishing boundaries with the external world, and dealing with the biological and developmental challenges faced by family members.

- It is not uncommon for developed countries to be the final destination of people who are displaced as a result of historical traumas such as war, genocide or oppression. This group also forms a significant minority among the vulnerable people who use frontline services. What is less commonly understood is that the impact of migration and displacement can be transmitted across generations to affect the second or even third generation offspring of displaced individuals.

- Sometimes migrants persist in using coping strategies that were effective for them in their previous milieu, despite these no longer being effective in their host societies. These unhelpful strategies can be hard to change and could influence the functioning and wellbeing of subsequent generations in ways that may not be immediately visible to practitioners. Areas that may be particularly affected include the family's relationships with the outside world, especially the authorities and those perceived as representing authority, and gender or family roles.

- Reflective practitioners are sensitive to the influence of family history and curious about families' stories and how past realities influence present behaviour and relationship patterns. They also reflect on how their own family histories affect their attitudes and assumptions regarding the services they provide.

FURTHER READING

If you are interested in the impact of geographically-based disparities on the health, wellbeing and protection of children around the world, the UNICEF report referred to in the text is a special edition of their publication *The State of the World's Children* published to mark the 20th anniversary of the UN convention on the rights of the child. The full report can be downloaded from the UNICEF website (www.unicef.org) and contains a wealth of information about challenges facing children worldwide in the 21st century, illustrating some of the points made in the text.

If you are interested in exploring further the social and economic impact of migration, the United Nations, World Bank, national governments and many migration charities have excellent resources available online.

If you are interested in the research on intergenerational trauma then the articles by Brown (1988) and Kellerman (2001) referred to in the text provide excellent summaries of this very interesting and substantial body of psychological and social research.

For further exploration of the psychology of intergenerational patterns in families from a family therapy perspective, John Byng-Hall's book, *Rewriting Family Scripts: Improvisation and Systems Change*, published in 1995, is a good starting point.

EXTENDED EXAMPLE 1

NARRATIVE APPROACHES AND FAMILY INFLUENCES

Danny is a second-year nursing student in a reflective practice group at college. The students have been asked to keep personal learning journals and to reflect on the impact their clinical placements have on them. Danny's current placement is on an orthopaedic ward in a district hospital where trauma surgery is a well-developed specialism. The following piece of reflective work starts with Danny recounting to the group an experience he recently had while on placement.

> 'Last Wednesday, while on my break, I saw them bring an African man into A&E. He was badly injured in a road traffic accident. As they unloaded him from the ambulance, I could see that his face was bruised and badly swollen. He was pale – obviously lost some blood. When I saw his face, something unusual happened to me that shook me terribly. I had a flashback to when I was 10 or 11 and we were still living in Africa. I remembered one morning just after dawn, hearing some noises outside and when I went to check, found my dad had been dumped outside our front door in a bad state. He had obviously been beaten and his face was bruised all over and swollen. One of his eyes was so badly swollen, it was completely shut. He was barely conscious. I remember the fear I felt and, somehow, mum must have heard something too, as the next thing I remember is that we had him inside and we were cleaning him up. I still recall how shocked I was to see the state he was in, but strangely, I was very calm when mum and I were cleaning and dressing his wounds. As I said, I was only 10 or 11 at the time, and had almost forgotten that incident, except for seeing that fellow come in with the swollen face just like my dad's. The regime's security people had taken dad three days earlier and after that beating, mum put her foot down and we fled the country and came over here.
>
> Anyway, having that experience really upset me. I went back to the ward and had to get on with my work like nothing happened, but I couldn't get his face out of my mind. The whole incident brought so much back to me – and also

about why I decided to become a nurse, I guess, to look after people like we looked after my dad that morning.

They brought the same man into our ward last Friday afternoon, but by that time I had recovered my composure and there were no unexpected flashbacks or strong feelings. I was just curious to know what had happened to him.'

Danny used this event as a stimulus for some further reflections which he recorded in his journal using a free narrative format rather than one of the structured techniques mentioned in *Chapter 2*.

My family story and my career choice

After my family left Africa, we came to the UK. For me the journey was exciting, but I guess my parents must have been very frightened for part of the way. Mum was a teacher back home and by sheer good luck her college had its qualifications validated by a UK institution, so she was eventually able to work in her profession. Dad was not so lucky. He had to take a job as a security guard. He just could not stop himself from becoming a champion for the underdog, and was fired because of his trouble-making. Then he did some labouring, and would always get into conflict with employers or supervisors, so he quickly became known as a trouble-maker. After that, no one would take him on. At home, mum wore the trousers as she was the main earner and I guess he felt ashamed at not being able to provide for his family. After about a year, dad took to drinking heavily and started convincing himself that the security police from back home were after him again and had sent agents over here to poison him.

We went from a family that saw themselves as part of the elite, with a professional mother and politician father, to a pretty down-and-out state. Dad was getting more desperate and delusional by the week and mum was desperately trying to keep things normal for us through working as hard as she could and keeping a sense of order at home.

As a teenager, I saw my parents as losers, and I lost a lot of respect for dad. I never brought friends home because of dad's paranoid ranting about security police and secret agents. They would have thought he was crazy. Dad never made any friends because the more he drank, the more he was afraid of being watched, followed and betrayed. And mum was always working either in her teaching job or doing some moonlighting on the side.

I always respected mum because she was a fighter and nothing could ever get her down. Even as a teenager, I always did what mum told me in the end, despite being very mouthy towards her. Mum and I took care of dad and would always sort him out when we found him after he had drunk himself into a stupor. Dealing with washing and dressing him and cleaning him up, while at the same time ignoring his paranoid mutterings, became par for the course and I never minded the personal care elements of this. In this, as in everything else, mum and I did what was necessary even if it was stomach turning and difficult. So I guess I took my sense of responsibility and coping with tough situations from mum. Every now and then I do feel dad's sense of injustice well up inside me though, and I get angry with the system or the corrupt people in it and want to change the world. So, I guess, my experiences in Africa and growing up in the UK, shaped my desire to look after others and not to flinch when I have to do some pretty difficult things that would make most people squirm.

It is interesting to think about how my life experience prepared me for nursing and predisposed me towards choosing this career. I am also surprised that this incident brought out so much about my history that I was not aware of in my everyday interactions.

Danny did a Johari's window (see *Chapter 2*) to summarise his learning.

Table E1.1 *Danny's Johari's window*

	Known to **others**	Unknown to **others**
Known to **self**	**Open** I enjoy nursing and taking care of others. I don't easily get queasy at the sight of blood or badly injured people.	**Hidden** I was aware of my family's history of displacement and what my parents went through, but pretty much kept that to myself. Secret shame of my family in the UK not shared with others.
Unknown to **self**	**Blind** I did not realise until now that taking care of dad and being responsible like mum influenced my career choice as much as it did. I am also seeing in myself dad's sense of right and wrong when there is injustice.	**Unknown** I never had the flashbacks to Africa before. Perhaps the extent of the trauma my family suffered has been kept locked away, outside of my awareness all of these years.

Discussion questions

This example illustrates a personal reflection from someone who entered into a caring frontline profession influenced by his personal history of trauma and displacement. Look back at the information given about Danny and try to answer the following questions:

1. Can you contrast how Danny's family viewed itself before and after leaving Africa? You can use the four family tasks given in *Chapter 5* to help you structure your thoughts. These were: developing a congruent set of images, evolving a central family theme, establishing a set of family boundaries, and dealing with the developmental and biological challenges they faced. How would you describe your own family's approach to these tasks?

2. Translate Danny's reflections about his practice story into the CLT reflective cycle introduced in *Chapter 1*. What sparked his curiosity and set him thinking? How did he go about looking closer? What was the transformation or learning that took place for him?

3. How can understanding the relationships between his family history and his career choice of nursing help Danny to become a more effective and reflective practitioner?

4. Consider your own career choice. How does your history relate to your choice of career? Can you think of a practice story where, like in Danny's example, events at work triggered something that reminded you of your background or life outside of work? Using the CLT reflective cycle, what can you learn from the events you described?

06

INSIDE AND OUTSIDE WORKING RELATIONSHIPS: BOUNDARIES IN FRONTLINE PRACTICE

CHAPTER AIMS:

The aim of the chapter is to examine the ways in which effective services are bounded at all levels and to help practitioners reflect on the ways in which the concept of boundaries applies to them. The material covered includes the following:

- Definition of the concept of boundaries;

- Bounded systems and frontline services;

- Service boundaries and how they are managed;

- Working with boundaries as a practitioner.

AT THE EDGES OF THE FRONT LINE: WORKING WITH SERVICE BOUNDARIES

This chapter is about boundaries in frontline settings. Just as boundaries and borders regulate the flow of people between different countries, service boundaries serve as barriers, entry points and exit gates within and between services. Service boundaries determine who gets seen, for what purpose, for how long, and by whom. Interactions between different agencies are regulated through service boundaries. As we shall see, boundaries outside and within services have powerful roles in shaping the relationships between service users, practitioners and organisations.

The concept of boundaries as applied to human systems is drawn from a theoretical approach to social science that is called general systems theory (von Bertalanffy, 1950). General systems theory takes its cue from nature, where every living organism has some kind of boundary that protects its physical integrity and regulates the influx and outflow of chemicals. Without such biologically active boundaries as cellular membranes or skin, organisms would not be able to function and life as we know it would not be possible. However, von Bertalanffy observed that there are similarities in the ways that systems operate, both within nature and outside it. General systems theory focuses on these commonalities between different systems and has found applications in a number of fields, including social work, organisational psychology and family therapy.

For the purposes of this chapter, we shall take a closer look at a single concept taken from general systems theory, namely that of an open system. There are many examples of open systems in nature, including all forms of life. Open systems take inputs from their environments and produce outputs that flow into the environment. Most human services can be characterised in this way as well. For instance, the inputs for a hospital diagnostic department may be people who are suspected of having certain diseases and the outputs might be the diagnostic evidence from the medical tests that were done with them. In a social care setting, the inputs might be people referred for social care assessment, and the outputs might be assessment reports and onward referrals. As in biology, general systems theory views the task of the boundaries of the system as governing or regulating the inputs and outputs, while the inner workings of the system transform the inputs into the outputs. Since there is such a wide variety of systems covered by general systems theory, this perspective is less concerned with the inner workings of systems (how inputs are transformed into outputs) than with the ways in which inputs and outputs are regulated and the processes through which different systems interact with one another through feedback loops.

REFLECTIVE ACTIVITY

Make a drawing of your service as an open system. Be sure to include the inputs and outputs of the system and try to consider the characteristics of the boundaries around the system. Mapping the inner workings, i.e. how your service works, is of less concern here than mapping out the inputs and outputs. Please make sure you leave some space in your diagram for further work as we shall return to it during a later exercise in the chapter. The example in Figure 6.1 illustrates what such a map for an IAPT (Improving Access to Psychological Therapies) service might look like. Usually IAPT services have fairly strict referral criteria with an initial assessment that determines whether or not they will be able to help. Discharge criteria may be more fluid, although time limits may apply to the duration of their involvement with service users. One of the reasons why IAPT services make for relatively clean examples of open systems is that the UK government initiative on which these services were founded targeted quite precise groups of people with specific problems with a prescribed treatment model and clearly specified expectations regarding outcomes. Things are not so clear-cut in all services, especially where services have evolved over time with changes in organisations' priorities.

Once you have done your drawing, answer the following questions:

1. Compare your drawing to the example given. Are the referral pathways in to your service as clear-cut as those in *Figure 6.1*? If not, are your referral pathways more complex than in the example? Can you identify who gets a service and who does not?

2. What is the process inside your service that people need to go through before they get help? (This need not be shown on your drawing as it is internal to the system.)

3. Is there a clear way out from your service, or are there possibilities for getting trapped in the system for longer than is necessary?

4. What do you think is the impact on individual practitioners of the way boundaries in your system operate? For example, do the boundaries of your service help to create a sense of shared purpose and clarity for team members about their roles, or do the ways in which boundaries are defined or implemented generate a degree of confusion and stress?

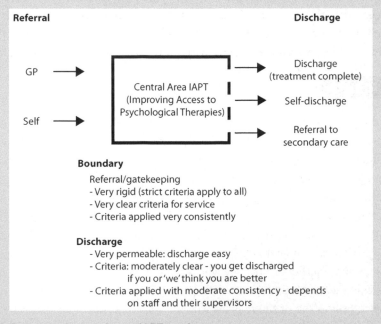

Figure 6.1 *Systems diagram for an IAPT service*

MANAGING THE BOUNDARIES OF OPEN SYSTEMS

Biological membranes have a number of properties that are important for their functioning and for maintaining the integrity of organisms. They are active entities. This means that the substances they allow to pass through to the rest of the system are actively controlled in order to meet the needs of its internal functions. Outputs into the environment are also carefully controlled, so the interior of the system does not lose valuable and needed resources and is able to get rid of waste products and other compounds that are unnecessary or undesirable to have within the system.

The boundaries around services serve similar functions. Depending on the functioning of the system within, boundaries can be permeable to different degrees. Services with rigid boundaries are very specific and inflexible around their boundary functions. This translates into rigidity about who is taken on and what is provided to service users. At the other extreme are services with boundaries that are so permeable that no one is turned away. Very few services can survive for an extended period of time with fully open boundaries. Even universal services such as walk-in clinics may have rules about service user behaviour that may go so far as to exclude individuals who behave in very abusive and disruptive ways.

REFLECTIVE ACTIVITY

Think about the ways in which boundaries are managed within your service. Are there clear policies and procedures in place to help you and the rest of your team determine who is eligible and what you are able to offer? Are you clear on when someone is ready to be discharged from the service? Are the boundaries consistently applied? To help you think through this, complete the two tables below, one for referrals into your service (gatekeeping) and the other for the boundary at exit (discharge).

1. Gatekeeping boundaries:

Place an X on the line to indicate how you rate your service on the following boundary characteristics.

Boundary characteristic		Description
Permeability (how 'easy' it is to get seen)	Rigid (strict criteria) ----------------------------- Fully permeable (anyone can be seen)	
Clarity (criteria for service)	Unclear ------------------------------------- Clear	
Consistency with which criteria applied	High consistency --------------------------------- Low	

2. Discharge boundaries:

Boundary characteristic		Description
Permeability (How easily does the service allow for discharge?)	Rigid --------------------------------- Fully permeable	
Clarity (criteria for exiting service)	Unclear ------------------------------------- Clear	
Consistency with which criteria applied	High consistency --------------------------------- Low	

3. Once you have completed these tables for your team as things are now, do you feel that there is an ideal state for your service that would be different from the current state of affairs? If so, how would your ratings in the tables above and your practice as a team be different under ideal circumstances?

4. How have the actions of your immediate manager affected your ratings in the above tables? How about other team members, other organisations, and your own contribution to the way the team works?

5. Are there ways in which referral criteria and formal procedures can be bypassed or circumvented? How often does this happen in your team and what is the impact on team functioning? What about procedures at discharge?

6. What happens to the boundaries around your service when the stress on the service increases in times of financial difficulty or staff shortages?

7. Finally, can you think of an occasion where the boundary function of your service had a direct impact on you? Try to use the CLT reflective cycle that we considered in *Chapter 1* as a way to reflect on and learn from this incident.

HOW ARE SERVICE BOUNDARIES REGULATED?

The previous exercise asked you to think about the boundary functioning in your service. What tools or mechanisms does an organisation have available to it in order to manage boundaries effectively?

Organisational policies such as formally agreed service specifications, local referral criteria, and clear and specific contracts with commissioners provide the official boundary around services. The quality of internal communication and organisational culture affects both the degree to which practitioners on the front line have clarity on how formal boundaries apply to them, and the rigidity with which the rules are applied. In many frontline services, clear formal boundaries such as referral and discharge criteria are well documented, but the extent to which these are formally applied varies, as might have been evident in your responses to the questions in the activity above.

One of the key tasks of managers at all levels of frontline organisations is to regulate the boundaries around the systems that they manage within the organisation (Zagier Roberts, 1994). A later chapter on team building explores the characteristics of effective teams which include clarity of roles and a shared purpose to teamwork, two team characteristics that are crucial to effective boundary management. A further way in which managers contribute to boundary management is through their role in supervision. New practitioners very rarely have complete clarity on how services operate. Management supervision has an important role to play in orientating new staff to formal system boundaries, but in many organisations, informal processes affect the ways in which boundaries are managed in addition to the more formal, rule-bound processes. What do you think are the unintended consequences of overriding documented procedures about boundaries in your organisation?

REFLECTIVE ACTIVITY

List all the agencies and organisations that your team routinely deals with.

1. In your view, who would be your main partner agencies? How do their functions relate to yours? Now add these to the drawing or diagram you made earlier. Be sure to represent what kinds of information and work flow between your organisation and others.

2. For each partner agency in your diagram, think about how the interface between your organisations operates. Are practitioners encouraged to have regular and frequent contact? Are the lines of communication formalised or are they based on practitioners knowing one another? Do you share information routinely? Can you do a table like the one in the last exercise for 'between system' boundaries for at least one of these partners? (It is possible that you won't know the answers to some of these questions. If you don't, it might be useful for you and your team to try to find out this information and share it, by consulting senior colleagues and taking the time to read your own organisation's policies.)

3. Finally, what happens to the boundaries between these partners when finances are tight or there are other sources of stress prevalent in one or more of them? Can you give examples of this and how decisions made in your and other organisations affected your team?

The following reflective activity contains a case study that might help you reflect on the issues raised above in practice.

REFLECTIVE ACTIVITY

Jane, who is 73, was seen by a community psychiatric nurse in the NHS, following an inpatient admission for depression. On discharge, the team did not refer her for a Social Care assessment, although her need for special equipment when preparing food and using the bath were noted while she was on the ward. On the ward, a bath seat was already installed in the bathroom and occupational therapy equipment was freely available in the kitchen, so Jane did not need special input by the Occupational Therapist. After several months of community visits, the nurse finally referred her for an assessment to local social services to address her equipment and social care needs. The allocated social worker felt that Jane should have been referred much earlier, but when she enquired why this had not happened from the teams involved with Jane, everyone apologised and told her that they thought about it at some point during their involvement, but with all the work pressure they had been under lately, it just slipped their minds.

1. What are the issues raised by this incident about the interface between health and social care?

2. If you had to locate the most likely causes of the problem, would you say that you view the problem as individual practitioners neglecting their duties, or do you think the fault is in the system, i.e. policies and procedures that were not robust enough to ensure that staff had to make an assessment of the need for a referral at some point during their contact with Jane?

3. What are some of the ways these issues can be addressed? Think of what the social worker can do. What about the social care manager and their seniors? And what can the NHS staff who worked with Jane and their supervisors and managers change?

This activity illustrates how easily issues that arise at the boundary between different agencies can affect vulnerable service users. One way that organisations can learn and improve their functioning is through creating channels for information to be passed between them. For instance, if the social work manager in the example contacted the NHS managers involved and shared the issues the case raised, it would be possible for the health service to address the root causes of any problems identified at their end, whether that is neglectful individual practice or weaknesses in policies, procedures or standards of care.

In general systems theory, such channels of information flow are called feedback loops. A feedback loop comes about when outputs from a system have been fed through one or more other systems and eventually end up being fed back into the original system as an input. Can you think of some ways in which your organisation has implemented feedback loops? Think, for example, of forums for service-user involvement, procedures to deal with complaints and compliments, and ways in which partner agencies formally relate to your service. It might be helpful to add some of these to your diagram of your system.

TEAM AND PRACTITIONER BOUNDARIES

The systems perspective mentioned above applies to systems at all levels of scale. In this section we will look at boundaries with our focus zooming in on a smaller scale, that of teams and individual practitioners.

REFLECTIVE ACTIVITY

Given what you already know about boundaries and how these operate, what are your thoughts about the boundaries of your team and also of yourself as a practitioner? Especially important boundaries include those around entry into and exit from a service and the levels of practitioner involvement with people. Are you as a team and as individuals good at clarifying to service users the purpose of your involvement and the criteria for ending the work? How do you prepare people for discharge from your service?

In my experience, many practitioners struggle to discharge people from their caseloads. This is often related to a perception of individuals as vulnerable and in need of protection as well as a view that appropriate support may not be available from partner agencies. Although practitioners may be correct in their appraisal of their cases, there may be other factors that come into play as well.

REFLECTIVE ACTIVITY

There are many reasons why practitioners hold on to cases longer than perhaps they should or longer than policies in their organisations recommend.

What do you think are some of the reasons practitioners find it difficult to discharge people from their caseloads? Try to think of reasons involving the dynamics of practitioners themselves, service users, and the ways that services are set up. Now compare your list to the information given in the paragraphs below. Which of the factors mentioned affect your service? Which particularly affect you? Are there any factors left out that you feel are important?

Service dynamics

Some of the most important reasons why practitioners do not discharge people appropriately relate to organisational culture. The organisation's narrative about service users may emphasise their dependence on the service and their inability to manage their own lives. A further internal cultural dynamic may be a covert culture of assigning higher status to those practitioners who work with the most long-term or complex cases, which therefore incentivises practitioners to hang on to cases. Poor supervision practice may leave practitioners without guidance as to when the work is completed and it would be appropriate to discharge.

Some organisations try to address discharge issues by making strict rules about the duration of practitioners' involvement with cases. If such policies are developed without due regard for the reality on the ground, practitioners may respond by not discharging cases as a reaction against the imposed rules (see exercise below).

A further reason for hanging on to service users is unclear contracting. People who are taken on by the service are not provided with clear indications of the type and duration of involvement they can expect. This dynamic may also mirror a lack of clarity from the commissioners of services about what is expected, which creates uncertainty among service managers about who should receive the service. Such a lack of clarity may percolate into every aspect of the service. Finally, people may be encouraged to keep cases on the books if managers within the organisation are inclined to defensive practice, in other words, to avoid complaints.

Practitioner dynamics

Practitioners may themselves find it very difficult to discharge some of their cases. For some, this may be about difficulties in saying goodbye to people who they have grown to like. Some find it hard to let go. People in the helping professions may have chosen their careers for specific reasons, including deep psychological needs to care for or rescue others. Due to their own attachment histories some practitioners find endings very hard to deal with. And finally, there are practitioners who find it difficult to credit those they support with the progress they make towards resilience, instead fearing that service users, once discharged from the service, will inevitably flounder.

Service user dynamics

Service users' attachment histories may predispose some individuals to fear abandonment and to experience endings as rejections (see *Chapter 4* on attachment). These individuals may have developed deep dependency feelings towards practitioners – a transference reaction that attributes 'maternal' traits to 'their' practitioners. (*Chapter 10* explores emotional transference reactions.) This may manifest itself in service users turning to practitioners for nurturance and guidance in areas of their lives well beyond the scope of the service. Service users with low self-esteem may feel incompetent and incapable of coping without the support and guidance of practitioners.

For many service users, the involvement of frontline staff carries a significance well beyond the practitioners' formal roles. Paid workers often provide social support and human contact to vulnerable and isolated members of the community. Loneliness and isolation may be greatly feared by service users, should they be discharged from a service.

Finally, some of the most powerful dynamics underpinning unhelpful 'holding on' can occur when practitioner, organisational and service users' dynamics interact with one another to forestall discharge. For example, a practitioner with a need to care for and nurture others may find it very difficult to discharge a service user who greatly fears abandonment.

WORKING TOWARDS POSITIVE ENDINGS

Working towards positive endings with service users starts with thinking about how different pieces of work will conclude, right from the outset. At a casework level this may include asking service users early on what they feel success would look like and how they would know that they are ready to be discharged from a service. By clarifying misconceptions about the aims of the service and clear goal setting early on, practitioners can ensure that they are always working towards an end to their involvement. The time boundaries of the work and distance travelled so far should form key elements in the agendas of frontline staff wherever possible and should remain part of the discussion with service users throughout the service's involvement.

A further casework aspect of the work is the quality of support that is offered by the service. Frontline practice can generally be viewed as either competence-promoting or competence-inhibiting (Booth, 2000). Competence-promoting support aims to respect individuals' strengths, reinforce good decision making, foster autonomy, and enable people to make their own choices with confidence. This kind of support is enabling and facilitates efficient discharge practice.

Competence-inhibiting support views individuals as incapable of managing their own lives, and intervention is geared towards helping them do so with the advice and support of professionals. However, the manner in which the support is given keeps service users dependent on the service. People who receive competence-inhibiting support may defer even minor decisions to the professionals involved with them. The practitioners, in turn, may actively maintain their dependency by providing succour to their wishes, rather than encouraging them towards more independence. This can be due to the practitioners' own need to provide care to the vulnerable or rescue the 'lost'.

At organisational level, good supervision practices will address issues of contracting and endings explicitly. Especially where practitioners' own dynamics make discharging their cases difficult for them, supervisors have a role in facilitating working through these obstacles to facilitate competence-promoting practice. In addition to good supervision, efficient and therapeutic endings are facilitated through ensuring that appropriate discharge policies are in place, and through making discharge planning mandatory.

Finally, reflective practice also has a useful role to play in supporting good discharge practice. When organisations foster reflective practice within all aspects of service delivery, the increasing awareness practitioners develop of both their personal dynamics and the dynamics of their service can also serve as a starting point for confronting and addressing discharge issues within services. As illustrated in the activities in this chapter, structured reflection can bring to light the importance of addressing the issue of endings in casework and help practitioners in devising practical and workable solutions for their settings.

A service has decided that all casework by its practitioners should take place in six-week blocks. At the end of each block there should be a review before any further work is done.

1. What are the advantages and disadvantages of such a system?

2. To what extent does this system address the discharge issues mentioned in this section?

3. Do you think such a strict rule would have any impact on how quickly cases are discharged in your service?

4. Now that you have read the material in this chapter, what do you think can be done in your organisation to improve discharge practice?

FOR THE JOURNAL

1. Reflect on an experience where you were the recipient of a service that had boundaries. You may have had a physical health problem, attended for counselling, or engaged a financial advisor. In the light of the material in this chapter, do you feel that the boundaries of the service you used were clearly specified or unclear? Were there ways in which boundary practice could have been improved? Now think of your own service. What are the similarities and differences in the way boundaries work between the two services? What can you take from this chapter to improve your own practice?

2. Make a list of what you have learnt about yourself, your team, and your service by working through the exercises in this chapter. What can you do to follow up on your learning?

Five key points to take away from Chapter 6:

↪ Within services, boundaries serve as ports of entry and exit gates, and as barriers to service. Boundaries regulate the interactions between different services and agencies, and they play a key role in shaping the relationships between service users and practitioners.

↪ Services can be thought of as open systems with inputs from their environments and outputs into the environment. The service boundaries function to regulate the interaction between services and their environments.

Service boundaries can be permeable or rigid (this refers to how easy it is for a service user to be seen by the service), clearly defined or unclear (referral or discharge criteria), and consistently or inconsistently applied.

- Service boundaries are regulated by managers in a service, and the ensuing quality of boundary management is a key task of managers and leaders in an organisation.

- When times are difficult due to financial constraints or other threats to a system, one common response is for the service to adjust the ways it manages its boundaries, by making changes such as devising more restrictive referral criteria or applying existing criteria more strictly.

- At a practitioner level, individuals also have a boundary management function. Experience indicates that in frontline staff, managing boundaries related to endings is a particular challenge – reflective practitioners cultivate their awareness of their own practices in this regard and use reflective processes, including supervision and team support, to improve their practice relating to boundary management.

FURTHER READING

There is surprisingly little work published about boundary functioning in frontline services. For those readers interested in exploring the concept of boundaries a little further, two useful books are: Hughes, L. & Pengelly, P. (1998) *Staff Supervision in a Turbulent Environment. Managing Process and Task in Front-line Services*, and Epstein, R. (1994) *Keeping Boundaries: Maintaining Safety and Integrity in the Psychotherapeutic Process*.

Both of these sources present helpful perspectives on boundaries within therapeutic, service, and supervision relationships. In this chapter we mainly explored the way boundaries function as ways to demarcate services at various levels and touched on how boundaries functioning in systems can include feedback loops. The two sources suggested here also include a wealth of interesting material on other functions of boundaries including an element of emotional containment (see *Chapter 9*).

07

GETTING TO THE HEART OF THE MATTER: HELPING PEOPLE CHANGE

THIS CHAPTER AIMS TO:

- Help you understand the process of intentional behaviour change;

- Review the stages of change model of behaviour change;

- Teach you strategies you can use within your practice to explore motivation for change;

- Explore strategies to enhance motivation for change and deal with resistance.

Have you ever tried to change something in your life, for example, giving up smoking, starting a savings account, or improving your fitness levels by doing regular exercise? Most people have, and, despite very good intentions at first, few of us succeed to see through all of the changes we would like to make to our lives. Why is change so difficult to achieve? What needs to happen for a change to be successfully made and what does it take to maintain new behaviour? These questions lie at the heart of the material covered in this chapter.

For many practitioners in frontline services, facilitating change is a key part of their role. The ability to reflect purposefully on why service users were unable to implement appropriate changes or, conversely, why specific interventions worked well, is a key skill for frontline staff. Being able to develop an understanding through reflective practice of where service users got stuck in the change process can provide clues to interventions that could help people overcome their obstacles to change. Reflecting on what works can help practitioners and services meet the needs of their target groups more effectively. Understanding the complex process of change will ensure that services do not subscribe to over-simplistic or blameful explanations of service users' failures to change. Reflective practitioners can place in context both their own roles in facilitating service users' attempts at making positive changes in their lives, and the points in the change process where people get stuck. This chapter aims to provide practitioners with a framework for understanding the change process and some tools to enhance both reflection on change and the practicality of helping people assess and problem solve their own change processes.

REFLECTIVE ACTIVITY

1. What kinds of changes do you ask people to make in your service?

2. In your experience, what are the factors that facilitate change in service users, and what prevents people from making changes?

3. How do you deal with service users who find it difficult to make the recommended or required changes to their lives?

In order to get the most out of the material presented in this chapter, it would be helpful if you had a really good example of an intentional life change either you or a service user had to make. This would enable you to compare your own experience to the theories and ideas presented.

REFLECTIVE ACTIVITY

Think of your own example of change. It could be a lifestyle change such as stopping smoking or any other intentional change you attempted to make in your life. If you are using an example of a change in someone else's life, make sure you are very familiar with the process as it occurred for that person. The change does not need to have been completely successful, but it would help if the person who attempted to change at least made a start at trying.

1. Map out how events unfolded over time. Start at the point when the need for change became clear to the person or to others around them, and continue until the change was successfully seen through, or until the change foundered. What were the key events relevant to the change, and what was it like for the individual concerned at the various relevant points in time?

2. What were the factors that facilitated the change, and what were the factors that impeded change or hampered progress?

3. What about motivation? How did the individual's motivation develop or change over time?

4. How easy was it to maintain the momentum of change and the change itself once it was made?

5. Are there things you can learn for your practice when considering this example? Think of factors affecting someone's readiness to change, forces that impel towards and away from change, and factors that help changes to be maintained.

Pete's 'Stop smoking' graph in *Figure 7.1* should help you get started with this exercise.

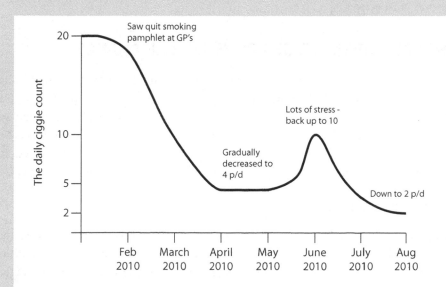

Trigger: Started smoking at 19 when a student. Hates the habit; there's nothing good about it; tried everything to quit, but with no success.
Saw pamphlet on help to quit smoking at my GP's & thought, 'I'll show myself I can do it – on my own'.

How it went: Managed to gradually cut down to 4 per day by willpower alone and it stayed that way for 2½ months. June 2010 I had lots of stress at home and at work. Went back to 10 per day again.
Managed to get my count down again to 2 per day by mid July but no further. I want to quit completely. To get from 20 p/d to 2 p/d by willpower alone is great. Maybe I'll go for some help or patches to help me quit completely.

Facilitating factors:
- Willpower
- Motivation
- Charting my progress
- Less smelly clothes, car, house

Impeding factors:
- Habit
- Stress at work and at home
- Social element: smoking with colleagues
- Addictive nature of smoking

Figure 7.1 *Pete's stop smoking attempt*

In order to understand the process of change, research in the way psychotherapy works and studies of people who attempt to deal with addictions or smoking cessation have yielded two very helpful sets of ideas; namely, the transtheoretical model of intentional human behaviour change (DiClemente & Prochaska, 1985), and motivational interviewing (Miller & Rollnick, 2002).

The transtheoretical model offers a way to understand how the change process unfolds over time, while motivational interviewing provides helpful perspectives on preparing people for making changes by enhancing their motivation. The rest of this chapter is based on ideas from these two perspectives.

HOW CHANGE WORKS: STAGES OF BEHAVIOUR CHANGE

The transtheoretical model offers a set of stages that individuals go through when they want to intentionally change a behaviour. This perspective therefore applies to changes that are under volitional control, in other words, changes we choose to make. Examples include smoking cessation, lifestyle changes, and any other change that the individual concerned decides to make. These stages do not apply to changes into which people are coerced, for instance, being ordered by the courts to attend counselling or a parent training course.

Stage 1: Pre-contemplation

During this stage, the scene is set for change awareness: Individuals become aware that changes are needed, but they have not yet consciously considered changing as something needed for themselves (DiClemente & Prochaska, 1985). In the pre-contemplation stage, a heavy smoker might become increasingly aware of the harm that is caused by smoking and some of the benefits of quitting, but there is not yet a sense that 'I' need to stop smoking. During this phase individuals' motivation for change may develop to a point where they enter the second stage of the change process. On the other hand, if motivation builds up and drops again before they attempt any changes, they may stay at this stage for an extended period of time. A key challenge for practitioners is therefore how to move someone on from pre-contemplation to the next stage. One useful method to assist with this is the use of decisional balance techniques, discussed later on in this chapter.

Stage 2: Contemplation

People at the contemplation stage are clear in their minds that they need to change. The general build-up of awareness and motivation for change that characterised the pre-contemplation phase has developed into a personal awareness of the need for change. Contemplators may be actively engaged with planning how they are going to implement the changes they wish to make. They might research relevant change programmes on the internet, read self-help books, or phone help lines. At this stage, the individual has not yet started to make a plan for his or her own change; this happens in the next stage.

Stage 3: Preparation

Once contemplators move from the realisation that they need to change, and start planning how they will go about implementing the changes they wish to make, they have entered the preparation phase. People in this phase develop a clear plan in their own minds of how they wish to implement their change.

Stage 4: Taking action

Taking action follows from the preparation phase. This may involve accessing services, trying a self-help method, or joining a support group. The person has moved through a general awareness of the need for change (pre-contemplation) to a personal sense of the necessity or desirability of changing (contemplation phase), made a plan of how to go about changing (preparation), and has started to take action to realise the desired changes.

Stage 5: Maintenance

The final phase is that of maintenance; in other words, taking steps to ensure that the change is lasting and steps are in place to prevent a relapse.

REFLECTIVE ACTIVITY

1. Go back to your example of change and consider whether the transtheoretical model with its five phases of change is relevant. Can you map the stages of this model onto the process of change in your example?

2. In your example, during which of these phases was there the most danger that the process would founder?

3. Think about your service and the kinds of changes in service users you work towards. From your experience, what are the critical points in the change process for them and how can you support them through these?

PREREQUISITES FOR CHANGE: WILLING, ABLE AND READY

In the previous section, we viewed the change process as a series of stages that unfold over time. One prerequisite for changes to occur successfully is the motivation of the individuals concerned. Without motivation to change, pre-contemplators may never move into the contemplation stage. Without a belief that 'I can do it', contemplators may never move beyond the realisation that they 'really should do something about it'. Motivational interviewing (Miller & Rollnick, 2002) provides insights into the various components of motivation and the processes that govern how motivation develops in individuals which help us to see how motivation affects someone's path through the phases of change discussed above.

Motivational interviewing asks two related questions: what enables people to change, and what stops people from changing? The answer to the first question turns out to be that people successfully change when they want to change, feel they are capable of changing, and are ready to take action:

- **Willing:** The person wants to change and believes that the change is important.

- **Able:** The individual feels confident that they would be able to change; feels they have the resources available to them so that they are able to change.

- **Ready:** It is important to change now, i.e. there is a readiness or sense of urgency about the need to change.

It is willingness to change that enables people to move through the pre-contemplation and contemplation phases of change into preparation. Feeling able to change through having the necessary sense of self-efficacy (Bandura, 1982), and feeling confident that the resources are available to help make the changes required allow for successful plans and preparations to be made. Experiencing a sense of urgency and determination that the changes needed are important provides the impetus for taking action and maintaining change, while taking action can be hampered by not yet feeling ready to change. As mentioned earlier, progress through earlier stages of the change process can also be hampered by factors such as low self-efficacy, or not recognising the need for change.

REFLECTIVE ACTIVITY

1. Re-examine your own example of change by considering the three factors mentioned in this section: willingness, ability, and readiness for change. What, in your experience, influenced you or the person you are thinking about to develop their willingness, ability, and readiness for change?

2. Can you list some questions you could ask someone to see whether they are willing, feel able, or are ready to change?

3. In the context of your service, what are the consequences of someone not feeling ready, able, or willing to change – for them, for you as practitioner, and for the service on offer? What courses of action are open to you in such instances?

While being willing to change, feeling able to do so, and being ready to take action are all crucial to successful change, the researchers and clinicians who developed motivational interviewing also discovered that there is a further question that needs answering; namely, what stops people from changing? (Miller & Rollnick, 2002). Before reading the next paragraph, make a list of all the factors that you have come across that stop people from changing.

What stops people from changing?

Many individuals in the contemplation and preparation stages of change find themselves in positions where they both want to change and don't want to change at the same time. For them to successfully implement changes the different sides of their ambivalence need to be addressed and they need to come to a point where they believe the benefits of change outweigh the benefits of not changing. When we discuss the decisional balance technique below, we will see that it is possible to bring the various elements in ambivalences to the fore and make them available for discussion.

A second factor that stops individuals from implementing even desirable changes is coercion; when someone tries to make you do something against your wishes, don't you sometimes feel like doing the opposite? 'Doctor's orders' can therefore cut both ways: for some it can represent permission to act differently or comply, while for others it may represent an infringement of their decisional autonomy, leading to purposely doing the opposite of what is required of them. A further consequence of coercion, however subtly it is applied, is that it breaches the ethical principle of autonomy and undermines the degree to which individuals feel they are able to make effective (good) decisions for themselves – hence coercion is a competence-inhibiting mechanism of support (Booth, 2000). This is why coercive strategies are so strictly governed in legislation around mental and physical health care (Department of Health, 2008).

A further broad reason that stops people from changing is when practitioners expect the wrong change. There is a danger that professionals who enter a situation based on incomplete or inadequate information may hold biased views of what needs to change right from the outset. These changes may not necessarily represent the best routes to desirable outcomes for the service users concerned. Instead of asking themselves why an individual is not motivated to make the expected changes, practitioners should ask themselves what the service user is motivated to change. Frequently an incremental sequence of small changes can lead to major behaviour change without the difficulties raised by trying to guide someone beyond where they wish to go. The next section presents a set of techniques that may help you to work with motivational factors in behaviour change.

EXPLORING MOTIVATION FOR CHANGE: 'WHY CHANGE NOW? WHAT'S IN IT FOR ME?'

Motivational interviewing offers a number of different techniques to explore and enhance individuals' motivation for change. In this section and the next we will focus on a small number of these that you may find helpful.

The decisional balance

In order for anyone to be able to change, the benefits of change need to outweigh the benefits of not changing. A decisional balance between four factors needs to be reached. These are:

- the costs of change
- the benefits of change
- the costs of staying the same
- the benefits of staying the same.

For change to be the most beneficial outcome for an individual, the following equation must favour the pro-change side:

$$\left(\begin{array}{c} \text{benefits of change} \\ + \\ \text{costs of staying the same} \end{array} \right) > \left(\begin{array}{c} \text{costs of change} \\ + \\ \text{benefits of staying the same} \end{array} \right)$$

You can illustrate this as the balance scales in *Figure 7.2*.

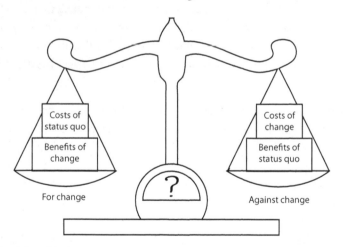

Figure 7.2 *The decisional balance*

The example of Nina, a young mother who, like Pete in *Figure 7.1*, wants to stop smoking, illustrates how a completed decisional balance might look. We will extend this example a little further when we consider the force field analysis technique below.

Nina is 27, a mother of two young children, and smokes about 20 cigarettes a day. She is considering signing up for a programme to help her stop smoking.

Table 7.1 *Decisional balance example*

Benefits of change:	Benefits of not changing:
I will be healthier	I enjoy smoking
The kids will be healthier	Social element to smoking
The house, car and clothes will smell better	Always felt like a 'grown-up' thing to do
I will feel better (physical)	My friends smoke
Higher self-esteem if I can successfully quit	I need a nicotine 'fix'
More money to spend on the kids or to save up for a holiday	Helps me feel less anxious
Breathing easier and voice less raspy	Gives short breaks from the children
Costs of staying the same:	**Costs of change:**
I feel under the weather most of the time	It's difficult to stop: I've tried before but couldn't
Expense of buying cigarettes	Irritable with the children
Worries about my own health and the impact of passive smoking on the children	Possible weight gain
Feeling low in myself as if I have no willpower; accusing myself of being an addict	What if it is too late for my health to improve?
	I'm not 100% sure I want to
	What if I fail? That would just prove I'm useless

Practitioners who ask service users about the different factors affecting their decisional balances can then proceed to work with these factors, looking at how to maximise those forces that will support the change and working on ways of overcoming those factors that are likely to impede motivation to change. One way in which this can be done is to focus on the discrepancies between the current situation and the desired one and ask the person how they imagine changing would help them. This is referred to as maximising change talk (Miller & Rollnick, 2002).

Force field analysis (Lewin, 1943) is another useful strategy that can be used with people who are in the contemplation and preparation phases of the change process. Individuals are encouraged to list all the forces that might support them in changing and also all of the forces that might prevent these changes from occurring. These can then be mapped out graphically and problem solving can take place around how to tap into facilitative forces and deal with forces that hinder change.

For the example above, the following might represent Nina's force field analysis:

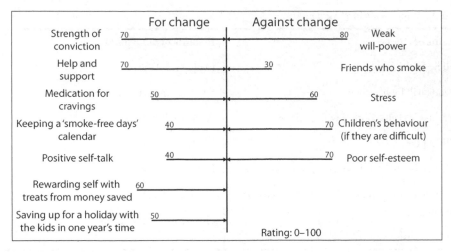

	For change	Against change	
Strength of conviction	70	80	Weak will-power
Help and support	70	30	Friends who smoke
Medication for cravings	50	60	Stress
Keeping a 'smoke-free days' calendar	40	70	Children's behaviour (if they are difficult)
Positive self-talk	40	70	Poor self-esteem
Rewarding self with treats from money saved	60		
Saving up for a holiday with the kids in one year's time	50		
		Rating: 0–100	

Figure 7.3 *Force field analysis example*

REFLECTIVE ACTIVITY

1. Try your hand at compiling both a decisional balance and a force field analysis for one of the major changes in your own example from earlier in this chapter.

2. How would you be able to use these techniques in your own practice?

ENHANCING MOTIVATION TO CHANGE

A key factor in enhancing motivation to change is the ability to develop in people a sense of the discrepancy between where they are now and where they want to go with their lives. Using the decisional balance, people can be asked about where their current actions are taking them in contrast to where they would like to be heading. Eliciting and amplifying change talk, mentioned in the previous section, focuses on increasing the sense that change can be beneficial to the goals of the individual concerned. This means that disabling self-talk, such as 'I can't' or 'I will never be able to' is replaced with 'I can' and 'Here is what I will gain from it'.

But what about resistance to change? Service users might get stuck in the contemplation and preparation phases of change. There are also people who try to change, and then withdraw from making further changes as things do not work out as expected. Intentional change is very rarely sustainable if it is coerced or inconsistent with individuals' own goals. This means that for some individuals, there is only so far that you can accompany them on their journey to changing their lives. For others, resistance may lie in feeling unconfident about the final push to living differently, or perhaps the goals initially set turned out not to be the changes the individual really wanted to make. Dealing with resistance therefore involves taking a step back and returning to earlier aspects of the change models described above: You may need to go back and work with the 'willing, able, and ready' aspects of change, or explore the individual's ambivalence and how they feel their sense of autonomy has been affected. In all cases, the best advice from those who have studied the phenomena of behavioural change is to treat resistance with respect and to respect people's autonomy, even if it means that the direction in which you wanted to help the individual does not turn out to be the direction they take in the end. Miller and Rollnick (2002) summarise this in the phrase 'roll with resistance'.

Finally, working with change involves more than working with people's goals or those of services. In a very fundamental way it involves working with individuals' capacity to believe that they can achieve something and live more fulfilling lives. And that is about enhancing individuals' sense of self-confidence and self-belief. Some of the techniques described in the chapter on narrative work in frontline services can be very helpful in this regard; for example, enhancing confidence and motivation through exploring those times in the past when someone was successful in making changes or those 'exceptions to the rule' when individuals were able to be assertive, make good decisions, and actively pursue meaningful goals.

FOR THE JOURNAL

The following questions might help you to reflect on yourself as a change agent: how can you use your knowledge of the material covered in this chapter to understand better where people who use your service become stuck in the change process? Do you see a use for the techniques introduced and if so, how would you use them and what would you hope to achieve? Finally, once you have tried to use either the decisional balance or force field analysis techniques within your practice, work through the CLT reflective cycle, focusing on how understanding the dynamics of change can help you enhance your practice.

CHAPTER SUMMARY

Five key points to take away from Chapter 7:

- ⌐ Facilitating intentional change in service users is a key aspect of the work in most frontline services.

- ⌐ Reflection on where people are in the process of intentional change can be very helpful in understanding difficulties in changing and addressing them.

- ⌐ The transtheoretical model of the change process states five stages of change through which people go in sequence when they embark on changes:

- ○ Stage 1: Pre-contemplation: starting to become aware that change is needed

  ○ Stage 2: Contemplation of the need for change

  ○ Stage 3: Preparation for change

  ○ Stage 4: Implementation of change/taking action

  ○ Stage 5: Maintaining change.

- ↪ When people struggle with implementing change there may be several possible areas where they get stuck. These include feeling ambivalent about the benefits of changing as opposed to staying the same, feeling coerced into making changes, or services expecting the wrong/unhelpful changes.

- ↪ Motivational interviewing is an approach that helps people to enhance their motivation for change. Even when individuals are satisfied that the changes they wish to make will be beneficial to them, in other words, they are willing to change, they also need to feel ready to change (timing) and able to change (confidence and self-efficacy). Motivational interviewing provides a set of tools that help practitioners to enhance these areas through, for example, enhancing 'change talk', working through a decisional balance exercise, and identifying the ambivalences about changes.

FURTHER READING

Many of the ideas in this chapter were adapted from the literature on motivational interviewing and the book by Miller and Rollnick (2002) is a useful and accessible introduction to the topic. You may also benefit from exploring the further reading in the chapter on narrative approaches (*Chapter 3*) as these approaches share a view of motivation and change that respects individual autonomy and offer ways in which to address change that feel respectful both to people and their processes, and a little different from conventional approaches to motivation and resistance.

08

REFLECTING ON WHAT IS REALLY IMPORTANT: ETHICS AND VALUES IN FRONTLINE PRACTICE

THIS CHAPTER AIMS TO:

- Introduce you to ethical principles and professional values that underpin professional practice in frontline services. After working through this chapter you should be able to:

  o Define the terms 'ethics' and 'values';

  o Understand the role of professional values in frontline practice;

  o Name the four key principles of ethics;

  o Reflect on the impact of policy guidance and legislation on shaping professional practice, especially in situations where ethical dilemmas arise;

  o Reflect on collective standards of practice and professional regulation.

ETHICS AND PROFESSIONAL VALUES IN FRONTLINE SERVICES

Practitioners frequently encounter situations within their work where difficult decisions have to be made with limited information. Should children be removed from their families? Should an emergency loan be granted to one applicant rather than another? Which of two referrals should be given the highest priority? Should someone be seen more quickly because it is known by the service that the family frequently makes complaints?

Within these difficult situations, practitioners face the complex task of balancing their personal views with the concerns and priorities of their employing agencies. If you have a professional affiliation, you may belong to a recognised body or association with published codes of conduct or ethics. These codes can provide some guidance regarding difficult professional issues, but ready answers are not always available for every situation. In this chapter we will explore the notions of professional values and ethics as these relate to everyday practice for frontline staff.

Defining ethics and values

Generally, the term ethics has two broad meanings. The first refers to a kind of moral philosophy which entails thinking analytically or critically about what is good, virtuous, or right within a given set of circumstances. The second refers to ethics as a set of norms or standards for appropriate behaviour; for instance, one ethical principle is to do no harm (Banks, 2006).

Values can be defined in many different ways, but in this context we will consider values to refer to a set of beliefs that people hold about what is worthy or valuable. Values are more strongly held than opinions or preferences (Banks, 2006). Values can be both personal and professional; for example, a personal value could relate to the morality of pregnancy termination, while a professional value could relate to considerations of social justice or integrity in professional practice. Your professional values are therefore those things that are important to you in your practice. This definition also implies that your professional values add a qualitative dimension to your work (Cuthbert & Quallington, 2008). Your values guide your attitudes, judgements, and ultimately, your actions towards people who use your services. Your values not only affect what you do, but also how you go about doing the tasks that form part of your role. Professional values affect what you consider to be virtuous or important; in other words, they affect what you give priority to. It is also worth noting that, while your professional values are likely to overlap with those of others in similar roles, they may not be identical.

REFLECTIVE ACTIVITY

Although there may be an overlap between ethics and values, ethical principles are usually taken to be more fundamental to good practice than practitioners' values, as ethical codes tend to serve as a norm for large numbers of professionals. For the following exercise, your task is to read the numbered statements following the vignette below and decide whether each statement refers to a consideration primarily of professional values or a fundamental ethical principle. State the reason for your answer.

Ethics or values?

When considering whether or not a child should be removed from a family, a practitioner takes the following into account.

1. Where possible children should remain with their own families.

2. Professionals should act quickly, otherwise it might be too late for the child.

3. Practitioners should not implement any interventions that might cause the child undue distress or harm.

4. Parents' decisions about their children should be respected.

5. Intervening in a family should make a positive difference, otherwise the intervention should be seriously questioned.

Suggested answers can be found at the end of this chapter.

REFLECTIVE ACTIVITY

As a practitioner you bring your own values to your practice. In this exercise your task is to list as many of these as you can think of. You can start by reflecting on why you chose the career direction you are taking at this time. What are the most important personal reasons for your choice? Often, these reasons are reflections of some of the values that you may bring with you into your role; for example, it may be very important to you that your job allows you to make a difference, help people change, and so on. In addition, some values refer to personal standards of conduct that practitioners set for themselves, while others are of a more general nature and shared by most practitioners in that particular role.

The following example, based on Banks (2006) contains some headings you can use as well as example values that a practitioner such as yourself may have:

Table 8.1 *Practitioner values (worked example)*

Value	Meaning	Example from everyday practice
Respect for others	I strive to treat service users and colleagues in other agencies with the same dignity and respect that I would want to be dealt with.	When invited into service users' homes, taking care to show respect for their property and family culture, for instance by not sitting in the head of the household's favourite chair.

Value	Meaning	Example from everyday practice
Autonomy	I respect others' right to make important decisions for themselves, even if these decisions are not what I think is best for them.	Continuing to support a mother regarding her child's difficult behaviour despite her unwillingness to leave her violent partner.
Accountability	I accept personal responsibility for my professional practice.	Not blaming a colleague in order to stay out of trouble if something goes wrong during a piece of joint working.
Integrity	My actions in every aspect of my work are honest and transparent.	Recording my actions in a situation accurately and contemporaneously, · even if there is a chance that I may have made a mistake.

Make a similar table for yourself, explaining your values with examples of your conduct from your own everyday practice. If you have the opportunity to work through this exercise within your team, it might be very constructive for team members to share their values with each other. What are the similarities and differences between different team members? Can you think of examples where differences in individual team members' values might have had an impact on their practice?

FUNDAMENTAL ETHICAL PRINCIPLES

Ethics as a branch of philosophy has developed many theories of ethical conduct which strive to produce general ethical principles based on overarching universal values; for example, respect for others. It is beyond the scope of this book to explore these in detail, but one approach to ethics, called the common morality approach (Beauchamp & Childress, 2008), has led to the following four widely used fundamental principles of biomedical ethics. These standards are frequently adapted by different professions when devising their own ethical codes.

The four fundamental ethical principles

1. **Autonomy:** This principle obliges practitioners to respect and foster the autonomous decision making capacity of people. For example, the Mental Capacity Act (2005) states explicitly that individuals with capacity to make decisions can legitimately make 'unwise' decisions. The same Act makes provision for individuals with capacity

to make 'advance directives' related to their wishes around medical treatment (such as resuscitation), should situations arise at some time in the future when they are unable to communicate or make decisions themselves.

2. **Non-maleficence:** Practitioners should avoid causing harm to others through their actions or interventions.

3. **Beneficence:** Practitioners should strive to do good, i.e. to provide benefit to others through their interventions.

4. **Justice:** Considerations of fairness and justice should underpin professional practice.

These four fundamental ethical principles are represented and elaborated in most modern codes of professional practice. However, individual ethical standards should never be applied rigidly as situations frequently arise where practitioners have to balance one set of ethical standards against another. The following exercise illustrates this.

REFLECTIVE ACTIVITY

Consider the following vignette.

> Joan is a mother with learning disabilities. She has a supportive partner who also struggles with learning, and a young son. Peter is a social worker in children's services who is supporting the family. Peter feels that Joan has a very good relationship with her son and that she is trying really hard to improve her parenting skills. However, she is making very slow progress and her son's needs are not being adequately met, despite a number of successful supportive interventions in the last six months. Peter and his manager meet for supervision and the discussion turns to whether or not the local authority should take formal steps to have the son removed from Joan's care. Peter is unsure whether this would be the best course of action and feels Joan would be devastated if she lost her son.

1. What would the perspectives be of the different individuals involved in this situation: Joan, her son, her partner, and the service manager?

2. Which ethical principles might come into play for Peter when considering the decision of whether or not to start the process that might culminate in the removal of Joan's son?

3. The Children Act (1989) states that the welfare of the child is paramount. Does this affect the likely decision the local authority will eventually make?

4. Do you think the decision might be different if the law enshrined the welfare of the family as a whole as its primary consideration? What are the pros and cons of such a position?

5. Either possible course of action for the local authority, i.e. to remove or not to remove Joan's son, could lead to conflicts between some of the ethical principles mentioned above. In this example, the Children Act states an overriding principle, namely that the welfare of the child should be paramount. What is your opinion on the impact of statutory guidance to practitioners on ethical practice in such cases? Can you think of examples from outside the child protection arena where such guidance might be helpful (or unhelpful)?

ETHICAL DILEMMAS

Ethical dilemmas occur in situations where contradictory ethical principles may apply. For example, in the vignette in the previous exercise, removing her son from Joan's care violates the ethical principles of beneficence and non-maleficence as applied to her, while such an action may be judged to be in her child's best interests. Ethical dilemmas are rarely straightforward to resolve, and very often a judgement is needed about which principle or party involved should be given overriding priority. In the UK a number of laws, white papers and other guidance have been issued by the government as guidelines for services in the public sector on the values and principles that underpin the way frontline services should be delivered. Where ethical dilemmas occur, the principles enshrined in these documents can turn out to be very helpful to practitioners when deciding which course of action to take. Earlier in this chapter, a few of these were mentioned. The following table provides a summary of some of the values and principles that might be relevant to professional practice in the UK from three such documents (there are many more).

Table 8.2 *Examples of value-driven legislation or policy guidance in the UK*

Law/guidance	Principles that govern practice
Children Act (1989)	Child's welfare is paramount. Making an order should be better than no order at all.
Mental Capacity Act (2005)	People are presumed to have capacity, unless they 'pass' a two-stage test of incapacity. People are entitled to make their own decisions even if these are unwise.
Valuing People (2001)	People with learning disabilities are entitled to all the rights and privileges of citizenship, including rights, independence, choice and inclusion.

1. Are any of the documents mentioned in the text relevant to your role? If so, how? Are there any other similar documents that apply to your service?

2. Together with some colleagues, decide on one or two of the most relevant policy or legislative documents to your service and summarise the content with specific relevance to the practice principles the documents establish for frontline services and present these to your team.

3. Can you think of an occasion when you were faced with a dilemma relevant to the guidance you thought about in this exercise? What was the situation and the dilemma involved? How did you deal with the situation?

4. Now that you are familiar with the content of this chapter, which of the fundamental ethical principles applied in the situation you described? How did the dilemma affect your values as a practitioner?

CODES OF CONDUCT: PROFESSION-WIDE STANDARDS AND PROFESSIONAL REGULATION

Trust is at the very heart of the contract between society and practitioners of all the professions. Over time many different professions have evolved sets of core standards and values that represent their collective attempts at being worthy of this trust, while society has increasingly demanded forms of enforcement and regulation that serve to safeguard members of the public from unscrupulous or harmful practices.

Profession-specific codes of conduct were mentioned at the start of this chapter. For many years, these have served as the basis for professional self-regulation. Self-regulation entails professions setting and enforcing their own standards. Professional bodies have formed structures that specialise in policing these standards among their membership and dealing with any complaints from the public regarding professional conduct. More recently, increasing political and public dissatisfaction with self-regulation has led to a worldwide trend towards implementing statutory regulation. This means that laws are passed which place the regulation of professionals under the auspices of independent bodies. In the UK, a prime example is the Health Professions Council which regulates a number of different professions, including Practitioner Psychologists, Occupational Therapists, and Speech and Language Therapists. The Health Professions Council may also take on the regulation of other professions such as Psychotherapists and Social Workers in England.

All of these regulatory bodies judge the conduct of practitioners against a set of standards or a code of conduct that combines professional values, ethical principles, and standards of good practice. Although the vast majority of professions have their own codes of conduct, taking a closer look at some generic standards that are included almost universally in professional codes can be helpful in understanding how these codes are derived. One good example of such a generic code is the meta-code of ethics of the European Federation of Psychologists' Associations (EFPA, 2005).

The EFPA code (2005) states four broad ethical principles:
1. Respect for a person's dignity and rights
2. Competence of practitioners
3. Taking responsibility: professional, scientific and social
4. Personal and professional integrity.

Each of these headings is then further elaborated within the code. For example, competence is expanded to include:

• Ethical awareness

• Limits of own competence

• Limits of psychological procedures

• Continuing professional development

• An obligation not to practise when ability or judgement is impaired.

This meta-code of ethics has informed the ethical codes and standards of conduct for professional psychologists across the European Union through shaping the ethical codes of their national associations, including the British Psychological Society.

In the UK, the Nursing and Midwifery Council have published their Standards of conduct, performance and ethics for nurses and midwives (NMC, 2010). The principles it states are as follows:

• Treat people as individuals

• Respect people's confidentiality

• Collaborate with those in your care

• Ensure you gain consent

• Maintain clear professional boundaries

• Share information with your colleagues

• Work effectively as part of a team

• Delegate effectively

• Manage risk

• Use the best available evidence

• Keep your skills and knowledge up to date

• Keep clear and accurate records

• Act with integrity

• Deal with problems/complaints

• Be impartial

• Uphold the reputation of your profession.

These 16 principles are further elaborated in the wording of the code.

REFLECTIVE ACTIVITY

Map the 16 ethical standards of the NMC (2010) code onto the four meta-ethical principles from the EFPA code. Are there some standards that fall into more than one of the meta-ethical principles? Are there some that do not fit any of the categories?

If you belong to a professional association or a regulated profession, do you have a copy of their code of conduct? Are you clear about the standards as they apply to you?

If you do not belong to a professional body, are you aware of any set of standards that do apply to you, for example, a code of conduct for staff formulated by your employer? If so, obtain a copy of the code and see if it maps onto the principles mentioned above.

Finally, if you do not feel any existing code of conduct applies to you, it may be worth obtaining either the EFPA or the NMC codes and reflecting on how you feel about the applicability of the different standards of professional conduct on your role. It would also be helpful to talk to your line manager about this as codes of conduct can be very helpful to practitioners facing ethical challenges.

In the UK, the Health Professions Council (HPC) also has a set of standards referred to as the duties of registrants. It lists 14 duties which more or less echo the list of the NMC mentioned above (HPC, 2006).

It is easy to get hold of most professional associations' codes of conduct as these are usually available for free download from these bodies' websites (as are the codes mentioned above). What differentiates one code of conduct from another is usually only a matter of emphasis or wording. However, reading several different codes of conduct may be very enlightening, as different codes tend to highlight different professional issues that are viewed as important by the relevant professional body but are often applicable more widely. For example, most codes of conduct emphasise that practitioners should not tarnish the reputation of their professions with the public. In order to ensure this, they require high standards of personal and business conduct related both to their professional practice and their conduct outside it. This means that someone who is convicted of a criminal offence unrelated to their professional practice may find themselves facing disciplinary action from their professional bodies, even though their work has always been of a high standard.

This exercise is best done in a group, although individual reflection on the issues raised should also be helpful to readers. Read the following fictional scenarios and answer the questions that follow:

> Jim is a student nurse and subject to the NMC code of conduct mentioned above. He was arrested during the 2011 riots in London inside a shop which was raided by rioters, but was not found in possession of stolen items. He was subsequently charged and given a community service sentence. The NMC has instigated disciplinary proceedings against him on the grounds that his conduct was unprofessional and brought the reputation of nursing into disrepute.

> Sophie is a newly qualified nurse. Last month she went abroad with some of her best friends for a weekend of hard partying. During the course of the weekend she and her friends were arrested for public order offences and released on condition that they leave the country and do not return for five years. She was surprised to find out on her return that, under the NMC code of conduct, she had to inform them of her conviction. She is anxiously waiting for them to inform her whether or not there will be disciplinary action taken against her.

Discussion questions

1. What is your view of the behaviour exhibited by Sophie and Jim? Do you feel they have acted very much like other young people in their subculture or in society in general, or do you feel that their behaviour was unacceptable under any circumstances?

2. What is your view about their professional conduct in these situations? Is it fair that they are held professionally accountable for actions outside of work?

3. What do you think should be the balance between personal and professional accountability for practitioners in your service?

4. If you supervised Jim or Sophie and were informed of what happened during their supervision with you, what do you think are the appropriate actions you should take as their supervisor? For example, does their employer need to know?

A final thought on ethical dilemmas: a key feature of the model of reflective practice that underpins this book is that reflective practitioners use their reflective skills to consider both the factual aspects of a situation and the emotional elements, especially as these relate to themselves as actors within the situations they deal with. In few situations is taking a holistic stance as crucial as in considering difficult and ethically challenging decisions that are made in services. There will almost always be an emotional impact on you as a practitioner when you are instrumental in the resolution of difficult dilemmas such as removing children from the care of their parents, moving someone into residential care who has become too frail to care for themselves despite wishing to do so, or placing someone in a situation where their liberties are reduced in order to protect them or others from harm. One of my hopes in writing this book is that, through your engagement with the material presented here, you will find effective ways of reflecting on the impact of these difficult aspects of your role.

FOR THE JOURNAL

This chapter's journalling exercise is to reflect on the ethical dilemmas that you have faced in your work situation in the past. To get you started, try to think of times when there were issues related to consent, professional boundaries, confidentiality, and the value (or not) of intervening in people's lives.

How did you conceptualise these dilemmas when they occurred? What steps did you take to address them at the time? Can you relate your thinking to the general ethical principles and codes of conduct mentioned in this chapter? Will you do anything differently now that you have worked through this chapter?

CHAPTER SUMMARY

Five key points to take away from Chapter 8:

- In the context of frontline services, ethics refers to a set of norms or standards for appropriate behaviour. The term also refers to thinking critically or analytically about what is good, virtuous, or right in any given set of circumstances.

- Values, in this context, refer to a set of beliefs people hold about what is worthy or valuable. Individual practitioners may have a personal set of values relating to their work. Professional groups also collectively espouse sets of values.

- Four fundamental ethical principles underpin many codes of professional ethics; namely, respect for autonomy, non-maleficence (doing no harm), beneficence (striving to do good), and justice or fairness.

- Ethical dilemmas arise in situations where conflicting ethical principles apply. Actions may reflect beneficence to one party, but may lead to distress or harm to another. Practitioners may find themselves in situations where they have to make difficult decisions in the face of limited information and under time pressure.

> ☛ Profession-wide standards or codes of conduct, legislation and policies or official guidance may help resolve ethical dilemmas, and reflective practitioners are able to make effective use of supervision and reflective methods to support their ethical decision making as well as the impact of difficult decisions on themselves.

FURTHER READING

The references to this chapter, especially the very accessible book by Sarah Banks, would be a good place to start if you would like to explore the theory and practice of ethics and values in social care. A classic text on ethics is the work of Beauchamp & Childress (2008), while a good starting point for readers who wish to explore their own values base in depth would be the book by Cuthert & Quallington (2008). Full references for these works are given in the reference list.

The codes of conduct from the Nursing and Midwifery Council (2010), the European Federation of Psychologists' Associations (2005) and the UK Health Professions Council (2006) are available from these bodies and also via the internet (see reference list).

Finally, *Chapter 12* of this book, which is on the subject of supervision, explores how good supervision can help you address ethical dilemmas you may face in practice.

SUGGESTED ANSWERS TO THE FIRST ACTIVITY IN THIS CHAPTER

1. Value – also a principle stated in the Children Act (1989)

2. Value – also a principle stated in the Children Act (1989)

3. Ethics – principle of non-maleficence (doing no harm)

4. Ethics – principle of autonomy

5. Ethics – Principles of beneficence (doing good) and non-maleficence (not doing harm), but also enshrined in the Children Act (1989) (To make an order should be better than no order at all)

EXTENDED EXAMPLE 2

BOUNDARIES AND HELPING PEOPLE CHANGE

Peter originally trained as a learning disability nurse, but after a few years in a community team, he changed his career to become a housing support officer for a housing association that offers accommodation and supported tenancies to specialised groups. He recently changed teams from their learning disability service to a team for vulnerable young people with complex health and social needs. He started a reflective journal to support his adjustment to the new role.

About six weeks ago, Peter's team was contacted by the police. They arrested a young man called TJ who was homeless, claimed to be only 16½, and had been caught shoplifting in town. The arresting officer suspected he stole to support a drug habit and alcohol abuse. TJ was from another part of the country and claimed not to have had contact with his family for over nine months, after he was kicked out of his parental home by his stepfather for his drug taking and aggressive behaviour.

Peter met TJ at a local homeless shelter where had been sleeping since he was released from custody on police bail. On interview TJ presented as a pleasant, articulate young man. Peter felt he needed multi-agency, multi-disciplinary help, including social work and psychiatric support. The local child and adolescent mental health service would not accept a referral for him as he was above the cut-off age for new referrals, while the adult mental health service indicated that he was too young to be taken on their list. Social Care told Peter that TJ's level of need did not score high enough on their criteria for him to be allocated a social worker.

About a week after first meeting TJ, the police called Peter with news that he had been arrested for a public order offence outside a pub in the town centre. Peter felt the officer was expecting him to come down to the station and sort TJ out.

At this point Peter started to become aware of strong feelings of anger in himself towards the agencies that would not take TJ on despite his very substantial level of need. He also felt overwhelmed by the expectations placed on him by the police service and frustrated about

TJ's apparent lack of willingness to change. The following is an extract from his journal illustrating the reflective process he engaged in:

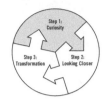

Curiosity

This case is really affecting me. All the doors from every agency I approach are shut in my face and it feels like I have nowhere left to go. No one wants to get involved. This young man fits no one's criteria. How can I help him? What am I supposed to do?

When I talked to my colleagues last week, two things became clear: Since no one wants to take him on, the police now treat me as if I am responsible for him. This feels very uncomfortable and also completely wrong. I would like to reflect on this some more. Also, given the latest development in his behaviour, I am wondering if he really wants to get his life sorted out at all. How do I know he wants to change?

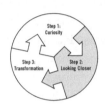

Looking closer

The boundaries around the different services appear to be really impermeable to a homeless person with his offending history. It feels like eligibility criteria are used to close the gates and bar him from getting helped by anyone. What is this dynamic all about? Could it be about practitioners and services being afraid to take on someone who is 'trouble', or could it be more of a reflection of other strains in the system, e.g. finances being tight? My guess is that it reflects our society's dynamic of rejecting those who do not fit in or behave in ways that are unacceptable. He is alienated from all societal structures: family, education, the law, and now he's homeless too.

When I think about the different services as systems, I wonder if there are ways of shifting some of these closed boundaries. Perhaps there are people in Social Services who work with people who do not fit the rule book. Perhaps they log unmet need, so I can feed his situation into their system of service planning. Another option to think about is to see if he qualifies for an advocate who can help him navigate the system.

The other issue is his potential willingness to change. I want him to have secure housing, psychiatric care, treatment for his drug problem, help towards stopping his shoplifting, and I want him to engage with support staff to help him access opportunities in the community. But what does he want? I don't know that. So, perhaps it's worth asking him what he wants to see happen in his life right now and what he would be willing to change.

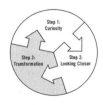

Transformation

Reflecting on this case has brought to light my frustration with other agencies and the system as well as my feelings of helplessness and anger when I feel there is little I can do to help someone move forward. I also wondered about what steps I could take to shift boundaries within social care. I will take these reflections to supervision next week. I will also take forward my thoughts about my own assumptions on the changes I may want for my client. When I next see him, I will talk to him about what he wants rather than try to impose my own ideas and see if there are ways to align what we as professionals want with what his perceptions of his own needs are.

Two weeks later, Peter has seen TJ again and also had his supervision session with his manager. He made the following entry in his journal:

Finally today some outstanding issues have been resolved. My manager attends a multi-agency panel for complex cases. Asking people there, he discovered a specialist team in Social Services for young people with chaotic lives and I referred the client there this afternoon. My manager also advised me to log his unmet psychiatric needs with local commissioners in the health system.

I saw the young man again yesterday afternoon and started to discuss his views with him of where he wants to go with his life. I was surprised how open and frank he was when I started listening to him instead of imposing the system's views. He was agreeable to a supported tenancy, attending college and getting help for his substance abuse, but qualified the plan in the light of his history and what he thought would help him.

He told me that as a young child he was always in trouble and thought he must be a very bad person, until he was diagnosed with ADHD when he was eight years old. He took prescription medication that helped him to focus in school until he was 14, but then the prescription stopped as his family moved areas. Not having the tablets and feeling out of place in his new school led him to try to obtain his tablets illegally through 'people' at his school. From there his level of involvement with drugs escalated and he went from illegally sourcing his former medication to trying other prescription drugs and eventually started taking a variety of substances as well as drinking heavily. His behaviour changed as his frequent use of substances took effect and he started stealing to maintain his supply of drugs – and it did not take long for his stepfather to kick him out. 'He didn't like me much anyway.' He got on a bus and left town, only to continue his previous pattern of behaviour when he arrived locally.

What he wanted was the following:

1. A re-assessment of his ADHD and a prescription or other help to deal with the condition.

2. Re-housing away from the town, perhaps in a rural area to get away from the people he currently mixes with.

3. Once his ADHD is addressed, he felt he would really benefit from treatment for his drugs habit.

We did a force field analysis that looked like this:

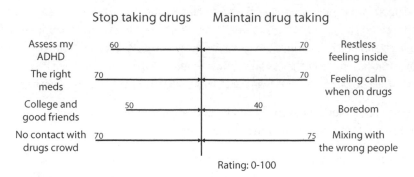

Figure E2.1 *TJ's force field analysis*

Discussion questions

1. Peter's first main issue for reflection involved developing his awareness of how to influence other systems and organisations. His initial attempts at making onward referrals for his client were met with closed doors as every service indicated that TJ did not meet their criteria. Largely by chance, he obtained information from his manager that helped him overcome this difficulty with one of the services he tried.

   What are the ways you have found that enable you to circumvent or cross rigid system boundaries? Do these depend on your network of personal contacts or your manager (as in the example)? Can you think of ways in which services in your locality could jointly address issues that arise out of their respective service boundaries not being consistent or compatible?

   Peter also fed information about unmet needs to his local health service commissioning team and advised TJ to get an advocate. Through making services aware of unmet needs and by engaging with advocacy, feedback loops are set up that enable agencies to respond to the needs of the communities they serve. His manager's membership of a multi-agency panel on complex cases is another forum where feedback into systems originates. What are the existing structural feedback loops in your organisation; for instance, are there places you can log unmet needs, or service user involvement groups? It is not uncommon for practitioners to be unaware of these aspects of their organisations, so if you do not know what is available, it would be helpful to find out. How can you use these mechanisms to support the development of your service?

2. Peter's work with TJ involved identifying aspects of his life he was willing to change. Peter felt that helping TJ reach his goals would make it more likely for the service/system to reach its goals as a consequence. Do you agree with his approach? Would that work in your service? Which assumptions that are routinely made about service users would such an approach question?

3. Peter originally trained as a nurse specialising in supporting people with learning disabilities. In *Chapter 8* you will find a list of the 16 main points on the UK Nursing and Midwifery Council (NMC) Code of Conduct. Which of these do you consider most applicable to the way Peter dealt with TJ's case? How do you think Peter could have used the NMC code of conduct to help him clarify his role and support his work with TJ? How would you suggest practitioners in your role use any relevant codes of conduct in their work on a daily basis?

4. This example contained excerpts from Peter's journal. What is your view on how he used reflection to help him make sense of his experiences? In *Chapter 12* we will look at case supervision in more detail, but what are your reflections on the way Peter used his supervision in conjunction with reflection to help his work? Are there techniques for structured reflection that Peter did not use but that you would recommend for someone who has a case similar to the example discussed here? (See, for example, the range of tools offered in *Chapter 2*.) Are there ways in which you could use a similar reflective process to the one illustrated here to enhance your own practice?

Note: As with all reflective processes, the example illustrates an incomplete and imperfect process: Peter could have focused on many elements of his case, but chose to reflect on the two most salient issues for him at the start of his work with TJ. Later stages of his involvement might focus on such issues as helping TJ re-establish a relationship with his family with the help of support workers to facilitate contact, or helping TJ get some help for his low self-esteem. These may well be fruitful targets for structured reflection at appropriate points during the case work.

PART THREE

REFLECTING ON EMOTION IN FRONTLINE SERVICES

09

ABSORBING DISTRESS: EMOTIONAL CONTAINMENT IN FRONTLINE PRACTICE

CHAPTER AIMS:

In this chapter we will look at the containment function in the relationship between service users and practitioners. The chapter aims to:

- Develop your understanding of the reasons why high levels of anxiety and distress are common in the context of service delivery in frontline settings;

- Reflect on how early relationships with caregivers can influence subsequent relationships with professional carers;

- Define containment and explain its functions;

- Examine the way in which containment functions in the early holding environment between caregivers and infants as an analogy for containment in service contexts;

- Consider some of the ways in which frontline services can foster containment in their practice to the benefit of service users.

ANXIETY AND DISTRESS IN FRONTLINE SERVICE DELIVERY

In this chapter the focus is on the relationship between practitioners and service users. At its most fundamental level, service users bring to practitioners some of their needs for medical, social, or psychological care, practical help or support. Their expectation, in turn, is that you will support them some of the way towards fulfilling those needs. Alternatively, your service may be imposed on their lives, making full engagement with you very difficult.

Examples of imposition would be when someone is on probation after serving a prison sentence, or referrals that follow on from child protection concerns.

REFLECTIVE ACTIVITY

How and why are people referred to your service? How does that affect their expectations of what you have to offer? Do service users' expectations match your own or those of your team? In fact, does everyone in your team have the same view on what you can offer to people who use your service?

The reason for your involvement is one influence on the way service users approach and use services. But this is not the only factor to consider. The premise of this chapter is that aspects of the internal worlds of service users also exert a powerful influence on the way they respond to services (de Board, 1978; Hughes & Pengelly, 1997; Kahn, 2005). In fact, there are occasions when service users present to services in ways that take practitioners by surprise because the ways they respond to the service do not reflect a rational reaction to the situation.

REFLECTIVE ACTIVITY

Consider the following examples of service user reactions to services they have been referred to:

> Suzi has recently been referred to Children and Young People's Services as concerns of neglect of her youngest daughter have been raised by school. The day after a very successful first visit by the social worker, she presents to reception at the social worker's office with a letter stating that her benefits are being stopped. She is furious, verbally abusive, and demands that the social worker sort this out immediately.

> Michael is a single father who recently started attending a parenting skills group at a children's centre. After the sessions, he regularly stays behind to talk to the facilitators. Recently he started phoning the office almost daily with requests for advice on small problems he has been experiencing at home. He has also asked the group facilitators for additional home visits.

> The Henderson family has been referred for family support. Despite sending a letter well in advance and phoning up to confirm appointments, family support practitioners have repeatedly arrived at the house to find the family out. On the last visit, one of the visiting

practitioners thought she heard children playing in the back garden, even though no family members came to the front door.

What do you think is the overriding emotion of the service user in each of the above vignettes? Would you agree that fear, anger, suspiciousness, or dependency are not unusual emotional reactions on the part of service users? What do you think would be the reactions of practitioners when faced with these responses from service users?

It is easy to feel attacked, blamed, and persecuted by people who react in extreme ways. It is also easy to encourage dependency and support people in ways that inhibit rather than promote their autonomy and competence (Booth & Booth, 1994). How often, in your service, do these emotions eventually lead to people being viewed with irritation, discharged, excluded, or moved on from the service?

Going back to the examples above, what do you think might be some of the reasons that the service users reacted in the ways they did?

As a starting point in our attempts to understand the strong emotions service users can exhibit, it may be useful to think about the extent to which the presence of frontline services in their lives presents people with a conflict. On the one hand individuals may find that their self-sufficiency and competence is challenged; on the other hand, the offer of support and its provision might elicit some very powerful dependency needs.

This issue is likely to be particularly pronounced in social work, family support work and related areas of practice. In health settings, service users may feel they have lost control over their bodily functions or mental faculties, which can arouse very high levels of distress. In settings such as the criminal justice system, child protection or probation, conflicts may be about service users' experience of authority and the intrusive nature of being monitored. The material presented in this chapter makes the fundamental assumption that conflicts such as those between autonomy and dependency, or between feeling judged and supported by the same person are relationship dynamics that first play out in individuals' families of origin. The manner in which such conflicts are resolved or left unresolved in our original relationships then become the template by which we deal with situations later in time that remind us of the original issues. In other words, the presence of frontline services in their lives has the potential to confront individual service users with some of their own unresolved conflicts. The strong feelings that may be aroused as a result could be a source of distress in themselves.

EMOTIONAL DISTRESS IN THE EARLIEST RELATIONSHIP

Psychodynamic theorists conceptualise these dynamics between services and service users by drawing on their observations of our earliest relationships in life, as these form the prototypes for all subsequent relationships (Kets de Vries & Miller, 1984). Our first experiences of dependency, love, fear, authority, anger and loss all take place in infancy within our relationships with our first caregivers. In the psychodynamic model, the emotional dynamics within our earliest relationships can either allow us to work through and resolve any conflicts regarding these issues, or leave us with unresolved conflicts that re-emerge later in life under certain circumstances. This same assumption governs the forming of the internal working model which we considered in *Chapter 4* when we looked at attachment theory.

All infants are believed to be born in a mental state where they are not aware of themselves as separate beings from their caregivers. Needs are expressed and when discomfort is not addressed immediately, the baby is assumed to experience very strong negative emotions – perhaps of attack or anger towards the caregiver (Winnicott, 1960).

The primitive feelings of the infant can be about immediate physical needs such as hunger, thirst or discomfort, but they also include some emotions related to an infant's survival instincts and psychological development. Fear of attack or destruction reflects basic survival instincts. As young infants start to realise that they have a physical boundary between themselves and the world (i.e. the skin), the integrity of this physical boundary becomes important. Later this may be reflected in fears related to the integrity of one's psychological boundaries. Over time, as the bond between infant and caregiver develops, infants start showing distress when caregivers leave their proximity. This is the root of a fear of abandonment.

Infants may also develop a fear of their own strong emotions. Very early in life infants are believed not to be aware that the thoughts and images they experience are contained inside their own minds. When needs are met as they are experienced and expressed, the only explanation for the infant is, 'I made that happen'. This makes thoughts very powerful, and it takes young children a number of years to move completely beyond the notion that their thoughts are not real, as any parent faced with a toddler who has had a nightmare would be able to attest.

When infants and young children are then confronted with situations where strong feelings are aroused; for example, by parents not appearing on cue or setting a limit by saying 'no', those intense emotions may be very frightening. From the infant's perspective, angry or attacking thoughts will translate into real attacks in the outside world. And these attacks may either destroy the 'world as we know it' or lead to retaliation which, for the infant, means annihilation. (Of course, such thinking patterns were originally inferred from children's behaviour and the fantasies they acted out in play in child therapy. There is no compelling proof that children really think in this way, but the psychodynamic perspective's value lies in the very useful analogies and clinical approaches this perspective offers, as we shall see below.)

In addition, young children may not yet have developed the capacity to hold in mind both the 'good' and 'bad' characteristics of others; in other words, they are unable to rationalise distressing behaviour by others. Emotions are experienced as pervasive and in the present (Winnicott, 1960).

When, for instance, an infant becomes infuriated with an adult who does not meet a need or sets a boundary, that caregiver then becomes the 'hated' object. The infant or young child may project unmitigated aggression towards them. But, from the infant's perspective, thoughts are real, and this implies that the caregiver may be destroyed by the child's 'attack'. For an infant, this arouses an intense fear of abandonment. Strong emotions can therefore be very frightening for infants and young children, but also for adults who have not developed the capacity to manage these emotions during childhood.

Although there is much inference involved in this account of early thinking, the notion that our thoughts can cause events in the outside world is not an unusual one, even among adults. Many people can relate to fearing that, on occasion, something unpleasant happened because of their thoughts. In the extreme, this thought–action fusion is a core symptom of obsessive-compulsive disorder, a serious mental health condition (Hyman & Pedrick, 2005).

These early feelings that infants experience are believed to be very powerful and also, in the earliest period, undifferentiated (i.e. the infant is unaware of exactly what the 'bad' feeling is about). The process whereby an infant learns to manage these emotions is believed to involve developing an awareness that the strong emotions they project will not destroy their caregivers, and nor will they be destroyed in a counter-attack. Instead, caregivers can take on these emotions and provide ways of managing them. At first, this takes place through holding and physical contact with the baby. Caregivers help to alleviate infants' distress further through feeding and changing them, and regulating their environments. These actions on the part of caregivers form part of the attachment process discussed in *Chapter 4* where we saw that caregivers who show that they are sensitive to a child's needs, available to meet these, and facilitative in terms of development, foster emotional security in their infants.

When an infant expresses distress, the caregiver processes the infant's signals (screaming, crying, physical agitation) and responds in ways designed to soothe, give comfort, or meet the infant's needs. The distress is alleviated and the 'bad' feelings go away. In psychodynamic psychology this is referred to as 'containment' (Symington & Symington, 1996; Winnicott, 1960).

THE FUNCTIONS OF EMOTIONAL CONTAINMENT

One way to conceptualise containment is to consider it as a process whereby the caregiver absorbs the infant's emotion, processes it, and returns it to the infant in a more manageable form; through receiving comfort, soothing and nourishment, the infant receives messages such as:

• No matter how upset or angry you are, I will be able to calm you down

• I may be out of sight or away from you for a small amount of time, but I will reappear soon and be there for you

• I can 'hold' your distress, I can make it better

• However aggressive your mental attacks, I will not be destroyed.

Caregivers cannot always respond instantly, but the consistency of their responses ensures that infants soon learn the ability to wait for relief and, later, to self-soothe, i.e. to be calm and alone for a while.

This provides constancy and the first steps to the infant realising both that he or she is **separate** from the rest of the world, and yet has an **impact** on the world. For both carer and infant, a mental model forms of the other 'in mind'. For the infant in the mind of the mother, the issues are about sensing another's needs and responding appropriately. For the infant with 'mother in mind', the issues are about differentiating self and other, emotional regulation, the ability to self-soothe, and the ability to make sense of the way the 'world outside' responds to 'me'. (Looking back at *Chapter 4*, this is the process of developing an internal working model.)

From this description it becomes evident that the abilities to wait, empathise, self-regulate, problem solve and think, as well as fundamental views of self, others and the world can all be located in the quality of containment in early relationships.

Containment allows the child to form realistic mental representations of caregiving figures: 'You can both meet my needs and set a boundary or say no to me'. It also leaves the infant with a sense that 'my strong emotions are manageable'. What starts as external regulation of emotions by the caregiver develops into an internalised capacity to manage one's own feelings (Winnicott, 1960).

REFLECTIVE ACTIVITY

Do you agree with the argument in this section, that caregivers' responses to infants can set in motion both helpful and maladaptive coping styles which can eventually affect people in adulthood? Can you think of examples where unresolved conflicts or fears that stem from childhood profoundly affect an adult's responses to other people or the world around them? Think of issues such as fear of being left or abandoned, a strong need for approval, or a fear of getting close to others.

Following on from the questions above, what happens when containment fails? Infants who do not receive a consistent, soothing and sense-making response from caregivers may find it very difficult to develop the skill of self-regulating their emotions. The capacity to think clearly when under stress is affected by fears of abandonment or other forms of psychological destruction. The sense of self is powerfully affected by caregiver responses in the early years, especially those that may have placed conditions on being valued or noticed. For example, what would the messages to a child be if positive parental responses were only forthcoming when the child made no demands on caregivers?

As adults, these early driving forces can underpin our basic expectations about ourselves, others and the world. Depending on which of the early anxieties mentioned above are most salient to the individual's experience, some or all of the following relationship patterns may emerge:

- **Splitting:** The individual finds it hard to reconcile opposing feelings about people or services. Individuals are viewed as either wonderful or awful, the service as fantastic or useless. Practitioners who are involved in both supportive and monitoring roles with families may find that their presence is experienced in a very persecutory way, with suggestions and advice responded to negatively as the family members struggle to integrate the two opposing roles and what they may mean for them.

- **Excessive dependency:** Individuals take on a helpless, dependent role, deferring even minor decisions to the professional and always seeking further advice and reassurance.

- **Projection:** Projection is a self-protective emotional response where an individual's own feelings are channelled towards someone else, or when feelings are directed at an easy target. For example, looked-after children may protect themselves from awareness of their feelings of resentment towards their own parents by projecting anger onto foster carers and social services.

In addition, some people experience an intense conflict between their dependency needs (fear of being abandoned) and their fear of attack, with the consequence that they may enter into a series of unstable relationships. One pattern this might take is to reject others just as they sense themselves starting to feel affectionate towards them and therefore becoming vulnerable to being hurt. Quickly moving on to the next relationship ensures that the conflict is re-enacted time and again. Another possible pattern is that of moving from one abusive relationship to the next, where the overriding feeling is that being abused is better than being lonely (Howe, Brandon, Hinings & Schofield, 1999).

Think back to the three examples given earlier in this chapter (Suzi, Michael and the Henderson family). Can you identify the key patterns involved in the emotional reactions described? For each of the three patterns described, can you think of an example from your own service?

These patterns all illustrate how early relationships may affect later patterns of interaction between individuals and those they relate to. There are many other ways in which an individual's inner theatre affects their presentation to the outside world. The essential point, however, is the idea that 'How I am with you reflects how I feel inside' (Howe, Brandon, Hinings & Schofield, 1999; Kets de Vries & Miller, 1984; Hughes & Pengelly, 1997).

People are usually unable to articulate their own relationship dynamics and the early fears these relate to (unless they have made considerable progress in therapy). However, observant others in their lives may be very astute in noticing the patterns. Practitioners, when regularly confronted with very strong emotional reactions in service users that are out of proportion to the circumstances, should consider the possibility that early relationship dynamics in the form of some of these early fears may be involved.

CONTAINMENT IN SERVICES

In the previous section, we have seen that lack of containment in early childhood relationships can return to haunt individuals in how they interact with others as adults. We have seen in earlier chapters that frontline services (and therefore, practitioners in frontline services) deal with some of the most basic needs of individuals in our society: survival, health, shelter, safety and psychological wellbeing. It is no surprise, then, that the dynamics of containment may equally apply to the way individuals relate to frontline staff.

If a service user reacts to you in one of the ways described earlier in this chapter, how are you likely to respond? Would you be able to reflect on those aspects of that person's inner world that may have influenced their response to you? Can you think of aspects of your own inner world that may come into play in determining your natural or intuitive responses? For example, how would you react when your offers of help or support are consistently rejected? Or to someone else's projected anger? Can you think of examples where the way you responded in the past made the situation better or worse?

Dealing with someone who is constantly aggressive towards you, service users who make multiple inappropriate demands, or individuals who become very dependent on your advice and support, can all be emotionally draining. The impact of experiencing others' strong emotions frequently forms part of the emotional 'cost' of caring. When faced with situations such as the ones described earlier, services make choices regarding the way they respond. For example, zero-tolerance policies may lead reception staff to call the police, should someone become abusive in a public area. Frontline staff may respond to different clients differently. For example, a very dependent service user's need for constant reassurance may soon elicit irritation in staff, which can ultimately lead to the premature withdrawal of a service. A service user who is suspicious of the agency's motives could easily be labelled as difficult or impossible to engage and face potentially punitive sanctions or premature discharge.

If you accept the argument of this chapter that, in many instances, the emotional responses of service users are reflective of their own uncontained conflicts rather than personal responses to their current situations, consider whether there are strategies that services can use to effectively contain these emotions. Can understanding the dynamics of containment help practitioners respond to service users who are very angry, excessively dependent, or ambivalent towards them?

I believe so. The secret to responding effectively to such strong emotions starts with understanding their early origins. Services need to give messages that parallel the messages that effective parents give to their infants during the process of containing strong emotions. These were stated earlier as follows:

- No matter how upset or angry you are, I will be able to calm you down

- I may be out of sight or away from you for a small amount of time, but I will reappear soon and be there for you

- I can 'hold' your distress, I can make it better

- However aggressive your mental attacks, I will not be destroyed.

Within the context of services, these messages translate into the following suggestions for enhancing containment offered to service users:

- Create a consistent presence

- Demonstrate the capacity to take on board and acknowledge the strong emotions that service users may present with

- Help service users clarify their thinking and apply rational problem solving

- Put in place clear limits and consistent boundaries throughout their involvement with your service, facilitating self-determination and good decision making on their part.

REFLECTIVE ACTIVITY

This activity is best done as a group role play. The role play should help to illustrate some of the principles mentioned in this chapter. In your group, act out a conversation between a staff member of a shop and an unhappy customer. For the purpose of this exercise let's assume that the matter of complaint cannot be resolved, so the experiment is to see how different ways of managing the conversation can make a difference to how both parties feel at the end of the conversation.

First of all, the shop assistant should try to be as unhelpful and defensive as possible. What happens to the emotional tone of the conversation as it continues? How do both parties feel?

Now repeat the exercise. This time try to apply the principles above. The shop assistant should ask questions of the complainant, acknowledge their feelings and try to listen to the complaint before responding. The outcome should still be the same in that the complaint cannot be resolved.

Discussion questions:

1. How are the feelings of the participants different under the two conditions described above?

2. What does this exercise teach you regarding dealing with angry or difficult people who use your service?

3. Have you made any observations about the nature of containment while doing this exercise?

4. Can you, as a group, think of ways to improve your service in the light of your learning during this exercise?

In addition to the steps mentioned earlier in the section, here are some further ways in which you can foster the containing function of your service:

Depending on your relationship with service users, you might be able to talk with service users directly about incidents where you feel you needed to contain strong emotions. It might be very helpful to your work with the individuals concerned to have a better idea about when and where they felt as strongly before and how those situations were resolved in the past.

It is important to ensure that people are clear right from the start on the important parameters of your involvement, including when, how and why you offer your service, your availability to service users during and after office hours, and for how long you can work with them. Talk about potentially conflicting roles such as monitoring or assessing versus offering support, as this can be a potential trigger for powerful early anxieties about dependency, autonomy and authority, as we have seen above. (There is more helpful information on the issue of service boundaries in *Chapter 6*.)

Promoting containment in your service or team

The following table provides an illustration of how you can analyse your service or team, using the points made in the previous paragraphs about containment of strong emotions within services. The information in the table is fictitious, but some of the points made could apply to many teams in a range of settings. How would the corresponding analysis for your service look and what can you do to improve your practice to foster better containment?

Table 9.1 *Analysing a service's containment function*

Area	What we do now	Gaps/areas for improvement
We offer a consistent presence.	Service users are allocated a key worker that stays with them throughout their involvement with our service.	We tend to use different key workers for subsequent referrals even if these come in very close to the previous piece of work ending. We don't match people to key workers very well – so sometimes service users and their key workers clash. We need a more robust system to allocate or change key workers.
Strong emotions are acknowledged and processed.	People deal with service users on an individual basis so this is inconsistent. Our team can be a little defensive when challenged.	Work on our own attitudes and think about responding in a containing way when we are challenged. Make sure we use our supervision better. Team needs training on how to deal better with difficult people. Practitioners need more support in dealing with very abusive service users or service users who behave in ways that arouse strong feelings in us.
We set clear limits and boundaries.	Practitioners deal with this individually – therefore can be inconsistent. Some of us tend to 'rescue' service users.	We can talk about boundaries more often in team discussions so we become more consistent as a team. We should design a leaflet explaining our involvement and the limits of what we can offer to service users and referrers.

Area	What we do now	Gaps/areas for improvement
We promote clear thinking and rational problem solving (competence-enhancing support).	The service expects people to become self-sufficient with support, but individual practice does vary.	Think about how we can help people think for themselves and make good decisions during our supervision and team discussions. We need to be better at closing cases. We need to accept that we cannot 'save' anyone from themselves or society.
We clarify conflicting roles from the start.	Very few of us clarify our support and monitoring function to people we work with.	Put this in team leaflet and make it part of our initial visits with service users.

How to contain a difficult situation in practice

In individual situations, containment consists of a sequence of steps which mirror the points made above about how an infant's distress is contained by a good enough caregiver. The process involves connecting with the extreme feeling, maintaining an active presence, processing and making sense of emotions and, finally, facilitating closure.

Connect with the distressing emotion

For both practitioners and services, the first step in the containment process involves connecting with the emotion. This stage is about not denying the value or validity of the distressing feeling. Even if a service recipient presents with an inappropriate request, the recipient of that request should acknowledge their distress and not deny its validity or the legitimacy of the actual feeling experienced by the person expressing distress.

In an example given earlier in this chapter, a service user presented to a receptionist demanding that she sort out a financial matter, clearly an inappropriate request made with an intensity that was out of proportion to the circumstances and the service's involvement. What would the connecting phase of containment consist of in this situation? The service user is certainly presenting in distress. The problem, to her, feels overwhelming and she responds with an attack on a representative of authority in general. Connecting with such an emotion involves the receptionist acknowledging her distress and listening to her story, which may be a little confused at first. Connecting to distress means not denying that there is a problem and not making light of the service user's reaction. Even though patiently turning someone away at this stage may be consistent with policy, this course of action could be counterproductive to resolving the situation.

Connecting with distress also means not rushing to the rescue, as that communicates a message of incompetence to the service user: 'You cannot sort your own affairs out, so I will do it for you'. This is sometimes referred to as competence-inhibiting support, as 'rescuing' service users or making decisions on their behalf which reduces their sense of being able to make good decisions themselves (Booth & Booth, 1994).

Maintain an active presence and facilitate attempts to process the emotion

The second and third phases of containment involve maintaining an active presence with the service user and their problem. Acknowledging distress and staying with the person through the process, physically and psychologically, communicates the message that 'we are not overwhelmed by this, we can help you sort this out'. In the case of the distressed service user mentioned above, this may involve the receptionist talking to the individual to clarify what it is they actually want from the service.

The process of helping individuals make sense of the confusion that they might be experiencing in their distress through listening, careful questioning and clarifying is a powerful mechanism of containment. The message conveyed emphasises that the individual's experienced and projected distress did not destroy the service or the practitioner, that even such strong emotions can dissipate and be made sense of, and at the conclusion of such a process, individuals may find that the solution to their distress is perfectly within their reach.

Sending someone away without listening or helping them think through their dilemma just increases frustration and anger, and also conveys the message that 'here we cannot or will not help you'. Sending someone away with clear thoughts and a plan of action they have arrived at through being listened to, communicates a message of respect, competence and the ability of the service to withstand 'attack'; in other words, the service is able to deal with strong feelings, even if they feel overwhelming to the service user.

Facilitate closure

The previous paragraph hints at the final phase in the containment process. Acknowledging strong feelings, validating service users' distress and helping them make sense of these feelings go a long way towards facilitating closure. Helping someone arrive at a clear resolution is the end point of the containment process. In some situations, this may simply be an understanding of how or why a service user feels so intensely in the particular situation; in others, containment culminates in a clear plan of action.

If containment has been successful, the distressed individual will feel they have moved beyond their immediate distress. Their reaction will be closer to a realistic response to the situation at hand. If containment has been successful, practitioners and, by implication, services will not have communicated an inability to face distress or a denial of their possible role in helping service users manage their feelings, even if there is a concrete problem they cannot resolve for whatever reason. Service users would not feel persecuted or frustrated by the service, despite the limitations in what can be provided. True containment also communicates messages of competence to service users, rather than maintaining a situation of dependency on professionals.

FOR THE JOURNAL

Use the framework given above to do a critical incident analysis on a situation you have encountered where containment was an issue and where the way things were dealt with could have been improved (see *Chapter 2* for a description of how to do a critical incident analysis).

CHAPTER SUMMARY

Five key points to take away from Chapter 9:

- This chapter took a psychodynamic perspective on the emotions that arise in the context of the relationships between services and service users. This view ascribes emotional reactions by service users to services and practitioners to the impact of the emotions experienced in their early relationships.

- The emotional dynamics that are mentioned include feelings related to conflicts between autonomy and dependency, power and submissiveness (compliance), and danger versus protection from harm. These are all processes that are relevant to both early attachment relationships and those between service users and frontline services. These feelings, when present in service–service user relationships, are usually excessive or exaggerated, given the circumstances.

- The way in which strong feelings are successfully contained in early caregiver relationships is also relevant to the relationships between services and service users. Successfully managing strong feelings in both of these contexts involves caregivers not being overwhelmed by their intensity, not responding punitively, providing a space to consider the situation reflectively, and some attempt at finding a resolution.

- When containment in early relationships fails, emotional defences set in. These include: splitting, which is the inability to integrate the good and bad parts of attachment figures, leading to someone being seen as all good or all bad; excessive dependency; projecting unwanted aspects of the self onto others, for example, usually intolerable emotions such as anger, fear and sadness. These emotional defences also take place within the contextof services and their relationships with service users. For example, service users may display unwarranted hostility towards services, idealise or demonise various practitioners, or become excessively dependent on the professionals who work with them.

↪ Containing a difficult situation involves connecting with the strong feelings that are present, maintaining an active presence, facilitating attempts to process emotions and providing ways for the service user to obtain closure. Closure can involve a number of outcomes, ranging from service users feeling that their voices have been heard, through to situations that are resolved through problem solving and making action plans jointly between practitioners and service users.

FURTHER READING

The book by William Kahn on the struggle to create resilient caregiving organisations, referenced in this chapter, is an excellent starting point if you would like to know more about containment and resilience in organisations.

The collection of essays by Donald Winnicott, entitled *The Maturational Process and the Facilitating Environment*, provides a cross-section of Winnicott's ideas about child development and the dynamics of caregiving in early infancy. Winnicott's thinking shaped the ideas of many later psychodynamic theorists about how organisations work and what happens in therapy. An excellent source of examples of how the early internal world of an individual can intrude into daily life is Patrick Casement's *On Learning from the Patient*.

10

WHEN STRONG FEELINGS MATTER: TRANSFERENCE AND COUNTERTRANSFERENCE IN FRONTLINE PRACTICE

THIS CHAPTER AIMS TO:

- Equip you to identify strong displaced emotions in yourself and in service users;

- Develop your understanding of the meaning and significance of these emotional reactions using the concepts of transference and countertransference;

- Guide you to use reflection to identify and deal effectively with these displaced emotions when you encounter them in practice.

REFLECTIVE ACTIVITY

Try to think of the service user(s) that you have most enjoyed working with. What were your feelings towards these individuals or families? What was it that endeared them to you?

Now think of your all-time least favourite service user(s). What were your feelings towards these individuals or families? What was it that made it difficult for you to work with them?

Chapter 9 looked primarily at strong emotions originating in service users where these reflect uncontained or poorly-contained emotions from earlier relationships. This chapter expands and extends our perspective by including transference and countertransference feelings, the latter being emotions aroused in practitioners through their work within services.

There are a number of factors that may affect how you experience the people who use your services. Thinking about the two examples above, can you think of some factors that determine your emotional response to the people you work with? How do these compare to the following:

- How cooperative someone is

- How service users treat you

- How your personal history relates to those of service users; for example, whether you have experienced similar life circumstances in the past, or whether you have strongly held personal, religious, or political views that apply to the individuals or groups concerned.

Experiencing strong personal feelings towards the people we work with is completely normal and happens all the time. However, it is also true that personal feelings can have an impact on the way practitioners manage their caseloads. Reflective practitioners continually develop their capacity to challenge their own assumptions and to think through their personal feelings about service users and how these affect their work. The converse is also true. Service users come into services with both their own histories and their service needs. They may experience strong emotions due to both of these factors, which is why services have, in addition to their function as providers of resources, support and care, a containment function (see *Chapter 9*).

We started this chapter by reflecting on some of the strong positive or negative emotions you as a practitioner may feel towards service users, and also mentioned the converse phenomenon; namely, that service users can come to experience strong emotions towards practitioners and services. In the next section, we examine this latter aspect, namely the transference reactions of service users. In the second part of the chapter, we return to the emotions that practitioners experience towards service users and services when we consider the phenomenon of countertransference.

UNDERSTANDING TRANSFERENCE

When service users experience strong emotions towards practitioners and services, these may stem from a realistic response to the situation at hand. However, service users' personal histories and the emotional load that is attached to their service needs can also affect how they respond to services. Depending on the nature of the needs met by your organisation, individual service users may literally find that their survival is at stake. For some, remaining together as a family, maintaining personal dignity, or recovering from illness or mental distress may depend on your input. It therefore stands to reason that users of frontline services may have strong feelings about the support they expect to receive.

1. What are the emotions experienced by service users when they first come into contact with your service? To answer this question, it may be helpful to think of the ways in which their 'survival' depends on your input.

2. Map out someone's journey through your service. What are the points in this process where these strong emotions are explicitly acknowledged or talked about? If such points in the process do not arise routinely, where can they be located or built into your service?

3. Consider your response to both of the questions above. How do service users' strong emotions and the ways in which these are dealt with in your organisation impact on you as a practitioner?

From the previous exercise it may have become clear to you that the stakes for some users of frontline services are very high. So high, in fact, that for many, survival in its various forms (physical, psychological, financial, survival as a family) is at stake. How then do service users relate to the services that are supposed to meet these needs? Psychodynamic theories hypothesise that when we are placed in situations where so much is at stake, we tend to revert to patterns of reacting that stem from early significant relationships (Kets de Vries & Miller, 1984; Teyber, 1992). In other words, if, in our earliest relationships, we felt secure, loved, and that our needs were being met, it is likely that, in situations we encounter later in life where we need others to support us, we will react with trust and a sense of felt security. If, on the other hand, our formative experiences left us feeling unsure of whether or not our needs would be consistently met and insecure about whether or not we are valued by others, we are likely to find it much harder to accept later intervention with trust; instead we are likely to revert to old patterns of coping and re-experience familiar emotions from these earlier relationships. (These ideas have been elaborated in several earlier chapters in this book, including *Chapter 4*, on attachment, and *Chapter 9*, on containment.)

What is transference?

When an individual re-enacts an earlier important relationship, such as that with a primary caregiver, within a subsequent context, for instance, in the relationship with their social worker, the relationship dynamic that they transfer to the new relationship is called a transference reaction (Freud, 1958). The next activity is an illustration of this:

REFLECTIVE ACTIVITY

Donna grew up in a home where her father was very domineering and extremely punitive when the children were disobedient to him. When she was referred to Social Services she was a single mother who had recently left an abusive relationship with a violent partner. She was allocated a male student social worker, Paul. In supervision, Paul mentioned that he found her a little docile and over-cooperative. After a few weeks, she started missing her appointments with him. The first missed session was due to a medical emergency with her child whom she had to take to the A&E department at the hospital. Paul only found this out as the hospital social worker was informed by the A&E staff that she had attended, and she contacted him the next week to inform him that the family had been seen at the hospital. Donna never phoned to explain any of her absences; she avoided subsequent appointments, and did not return his phone calls.

Questions for discussion:

1. What was Donna's likely reaction as a child to her father's punitive behaviour?

2. What reaction did she expect from Paul about her non-attendance, given her relationship history with males? What would have been her emotions in response to this expectation?

3. What do you think could be some of the reasons she did not return Paul's calls or attend further appointments? How would a transference reaction explain her behaviour?

4. How do you think a service like yours would respond to a similar situation? How do you think the service should respond?

One of the key characteristics of transference feelings is that they do not represent the reality of the relationship within which they arise. In the above example, Donna's feelings towards Paul as a male may have been triggered by her not being able to attend an appointment due to unforeseen circumstances.

Her history with males in authority, such as her father, may have predisposed her to expect the same punitive reaction she experienced from her father as a child in Paul's response to her non-attendance, irrespective of whether Paul gave her any cause to believe that he would react in this way.

Transference reactions are almost always unrelated to a realistic appraisal of the situation at hand, although, in cases of significant similarities (perhaps Paul did give her cause to believe he would react punitively to a missed appointment), these reactions are usually out of proportion to the situation that elicited them.

A second feature of transference reactions is that they tend to reflect the individual's own core psychological conflicts, especially those that arose in key early relationships such as the relationship with caregivers. For Donna, in the example above, her feelings, possibly of shame and fear when faced with a father in a rage, may have been so strong that she felt paralysed and could not act to let Paul know about what had happened. For fear of his expected punitive reaction, she may have avoided contact with him afterwards. These reactions stem from childhood and were elicited because Donna's 'inner theatre' played out her early childhood relationship in the present, without reference to whether or not her reactions were reasonable responses to the situation at hand.

Identifying and managing transference reactions

Identifying a transference reaction in a service user is not easy; however, here are some clues that might help:

- Transference reactions are often intense emotions that are out of kilter with the circumstances in which they arise.

- They reflect responses that may have been prevalent or appropriate in earlier key relationships, but are not helpful in the current context. It is not unusual for a transference reaction to centre on an unresolved emotional conflict from the past.

- Practitioners often experience these reactions as puzzling and somehow excessive, given the circumstances. For example, service users may be angry or hostile, no matter how benign the service's involvement. Alternatively, an individual may be excessively dependent on a team or practitioner, or idolise someone in the service.

Once you have become aware of a potential transference reaction in a service user, it is important to make an attempt to understand what the emotion is all about. Reflection with others in your team or taking your hunch to supervision may be helpful steps. It is tempting to try to manage all transference reactions in service users through confrontation and open discussion, but this may not always be the most appropriate course of action. Transference reactions often reflect very deep seated psychological conflicts which individuals may not be aware of. While you may well be correct in identifying a response as a transference reaction, the individual concerned may not be psychologically ready to deal with the conflict you might expose by confronting their reaction. Practitioners should also always be aware that they may be wrong about the person. For example, in the practice example above, Donna may have correctly inferred that Paul's reaction to her non-attendance would be punitive. Through reflective practice and good supervision, Paul may be fortunate enough to recognise this and deal with an issue of his that was brought to the fore by the way Donna responded to him.

REFLECTIVE ACTIVITY

This activity will work best if done in the form of a group discussion, although individuals can also benefit from working through the exercise. The following list presents a variety of methods for dealing with transference reactions in service users. Your task is to select the method(s) you think most appropriate to each of the case vignettes from the list below. In all cases it is assumed that the practitioners involved will get supervision on their casework.

1. **Call the reaction:** Confront the person with your view that their reaction is not about you or the here and now, but about another relationship from their past.

2. **Talk about the significance of the person's emotions:** Discuss with the person the significance of their emotions and how their early relationships are affecting their present relationships.

3. **Set boundaries, clarify limits:** Make clear to the person where the boundaries of your involvement lie.

4. **Set boundaries, clarify expectations:** Make clear to the person what your role is and how you can help them, and also what is expected of them by the service.

5. **Consistency of approach across team members:** Ensure that the whole team is aware of what is happening and able to respond consistently to the person.

6. **Discuss in supervision:** Discuss the situation in supervision, but do nothing else for a period of 'watchful waiting'.

Vignettes

a) Jenny is a social worker just starting a carer's assessment with Sarah, a young single mother of a disabled child who spent several years in care herself. There are no child protection concerns. Sarah's reaction to Jenny has been one of anger and hostility, including an accusation that Jenny is just waiting for her to make a mistake with her son, so she can remove him from her care.

b) Daren is a family support worker, supporting Amy and Steven, a young couple with two children. Amy phones Daren at least twice a day asking him for advice on minor management issues with the children. It appears to Daren as if she is unable to make any decisions for herself.

c) Tamisha is a support worker for a housing association. She has recently started to support Ashley, a young person who used to be homeless. Ashley has few friends and constantly visits the office, asking for help with decisions and issues that fall beyond Tamisha's remit. Ashley recently told the receptionist that Tamisha has saved her life and she wants to become a support worker too.

d) Chris is a care worker in a children's home. One of the boys keeps following him around asking him to take him home and adopt him.

There are no right or wrong answers to the best ways of approaching the situations in these vignettes. However, formulating the reasons why you favour a certain course of action and role playing the conversations with service users or supervisors that may arise for practitioners facing such situations can be very helpful in understanding how to deal with transference reactions. My suggested answers are given at the end of the chapter.

A final word about transference reactions – it is often very tempting to attribute any apparently irrational reaction by a service user to their own internal dynamics. This may absolve practitioners and teams from accepting responsibility for their role in their relationships with service users. Although transference reactions are very valuable explanations for individuals' behaviour, service users may have strong, legitimate emotions about the services they use. For example, a service or department may well appear to be very rigid and bureaucratic to people who attend and consequently elicit legitimate frustration or anger. As you develop your reflective skills, you should constantly question your own assumptions and continually look both inwards (at yourself) and outwards (at your service) to find explanations for behaviour you find confusing or out of proportion to the circumstances.

COUNTERTRANSFERENCE – WHY MY FEELINGS MATTER

Due to the nature of the work in frontline settings, it is almost impossible to avoid responding with emotion to the work. Relationships with service users and colleagues, feelings about the service itself and the demands made on staff, as well as strong feelings about the relationships between different services and agencies involved with service users are all common sources of emotional reactions in practitioners.

What is countertransference?

The feelings that practitioners develop in the context of their work environment can be understandable in the light of the situations they encounter and proportionate to the circumstances. However, this is not always the case. Whereas transference reactions in service users represent the displacement of emotions that characterised earlier key relationships into current relationships, countertransference emotions are emotions that practitioners bring into their relationships with service users from their (i.e. the practitioners') past key relationships (Berne, 1975; Teyber, 1992). These feelings share the core features of transference feelings, namely, that they are out of proportion to the situation at hand and that they reflect earlier relationship dynamics in the lives of practitioners.

In some situations, countertransference feelings in practitioners can be so intense that they prevent them from managing their work in a professional manner and therefore affect fitness to practice. More common, though, are reactions that are intense enough to be noticeable to a self-aware and reflective practitioner, but not so intense as to be detrimental to professional practice.

Countertransference reactions that fall in the latter category provide fertile ground for practitioners to explore their own emotional dynamics as these relate to their work. Countertransference reactions may also provide clues that lead to useful clinical information if managed appropriately. The following exercise invites you to explore examples of countertransference feelings.

REFLECTIVE ACTIVITY

1. List some work situations that you think may elicit powerful countertransference feelings in the following practitioners:

   a. Ann is a nurse who lost her mother to breast cancer when she was 11.

   b. Gemma is a play therapist who, as a child, was strongly affected by the breakup of her parents' marriage, which came about after it emerged that her mother had had an affair with a close friend of her father.

   c. Henk is a care worker who spent time in care himself.

   d. Gloria fled her home country after her ethnic group was subject to persecution. She now works as a family support worker in a children's centre in a multi-ethnic community.

2. Can you think of some examples where practitioners in your role may be at risk of countertransference reactions, either due to their personal histories or some of their attitudes or beliefs?

3. Have you experienced work situations where you had strong emotional reactions during a piece of work that, in retrospect, were countertransference feelings? How did you deal with these?

As is evident in the examples from the previous exercise, countertransference reactions can be a hindrance to professional practice. When your emotional reactions prevent you from working effectively and empathically with your clients, professional responsibility requires that you seek supervision to deal with the issues concerned. A fairly straightforward example is when your clients elicit reactions in you based on similar experiences you may have had in your distant or recent past. This does not disqualify you from working with such clients, but it is important that you are aware of your reactions, seek supervision, support and professional help if needed, and reflect honestly and openly about the impact on your work.

Your ability to manage your own emotions may be affected if you are under stress yourself. When we are fatigued or under strain, our capacity to contain others' emotions is reduced and our judgement may also be affected. Self-awareness and good supervision are keys to responsible practice in these situations. Sometimes it is better not to work with certain clients until you feel you are able to offer the containment needed. The exercises in *Chapter 13* on stress and burnout provide a starting point for recognising when you may need to seek further support.

Can countertransference reactions be helpful?

It may seem from the previous section that these emotions are almost always destructive and interfering. However, reflective, self-aware practitioners may be able to use their emotional reactions as a source of helpful intuitive information that could serve to help them understand better the people they serve. For example, the sense of futility and confusion you might feel after an interview with a mother who suffers from postnatal depression might tell you something about what it feels like for her to be overwhelmed by the demands of motherhood. Your confusion about the case may reflect her difficulty with clear thinking and making decisions as she attempts to manage daily life, while feeling overwhelmed and isolated.

Consequently, countertransference reactions, although they belong to you, can be immensely helpful in progressing work with complex clients. As you become more experienced at reflecting on your own reactions, you might also experience a keener ability to discern your own countertransference reactions and what they might mean for your casework. The following exercise invites you to explore a hypothetical countertransference reaction with the aim of developing useful hypotheses.

REFLECTIVE ACTIVITY

You find yourself getting very irritated with a service user who keeps asking for your advice on, and support with minor issues that are only marginally related to your remit.

Have you come across such a situation in your work role? If so, how did you deal with it?

Now think about your reaction in the hypothetical scenario above. What does your reaction tell you about the likely reactions of other professionals to this person? How would the emotional reactions of professionals affect the judgements they make about someone and their approach to their cases? What do you think could be some of the issues for the service user that lead to this kind of response to professionals? What might be some issues for professionals that might lead to this response to service users? How might understanding your emotional reaction to a service user help you in managing the case?

You should note that countertransference reactions are not invariably negative towards service users. Positive countertransference reactions also occur frequently and have similar implications for practice, both positive and negative. The following examples illustrate this:

Petra is a family support practitioner. She started working with Alice, a young single mother, two years ago. Initially she intended to do a piece of work around boundary setting with Alice. Since starting the initial piece of work with her, she never seriously considered discharging Alice, despite the service having a policy of reviewing work every six weeks. When recently asked by a new manager in supervision why the case is still open, Petra found herself feeling very worried that Alice would not cope without her support.

Shaun started work with looked-after children as a residential carer about six months ago. He keeps finding himself becoming emotionally drawn to Eric, a young person in the home who comes from the same estate Shaun grew up in. He often wishes he could take Eric home with him to introduce him to his family.

In these examples, the background information given on the practitioners is not sufficient to explain their emotional reactions. If you have to infer possible reasons why they might have reacted to the service users in the ways described, what might those reasons be? (If you are part of a group, perhaps your group members can role play a supervision session where one of the scenarios is explored by a case worker and their supervisor.) Assuming that the reactions described are indeed countertransference reactions, in what ways do you think they are detrimental to helping the service users? In what ways can these reactions be utilised to support effective service provision?

When can countertransference reactions be helpful and when do they hinder?

The following lists may help you discern when countertransference reactions can be helpful and when these reactions are detrimental to your practice.

When can countertransference be helpful?

1. When we can use our reactions to help guide us in understanding service users better.
2. When we can use our reactions to reflect on what is happening in the relationship between practitioners and service users. For example, these feelings often alert us to process issues for practitioners such as difficulties dealing with loss, a fear of confrontation, resentment of service users in the face of a lack of appreciation for help rendered, and practitioner responses to feedback or criticism.
3. When we are able to feed our reaction back to service users as an intervention to help them move forward, e.g. 'When I started working with you I was really aware of your anger, and even a little afraid at times, but that has changed now as I got to know you better. Have you had this impact on others as well? I wonder what the impact of that might have been on relationships with others you had in the past?'

When does countertransference get in the way of providing effective support?

1. When it is not recognised and dealt with. Sometimes dealing with countertransference means just being aware for yourself and making sure that your own emotions do not get in the way of providing an effective service.
2. When it becomes such a strong reaction on your part that you can't work effectively with someone.
3. When your countertransference reactions prevent you from doing the work. For example, there could be collusion between practitioners and service users to avoid dealing with something that is difficult for both of them to face; for instance, a practitioner who fears confrontation may not bring into the open a service user's strong feelings of anger at the service. This may deny the service user an opportunity to learn about the impact of their behaviour on others, the service may not get useful feedback, and the service may fail in its containment function (as discussed in *Chapter 9*).

How should countertransference reactions be managed?

The process starts with awareness. As a practitioner, you need to remain alert to the possibility that your emotional reaction to a situation you encounter in the course of your work, may reflect an aspect of your personal history that is as yet unresolved. Ask yourself regularly, 'How do I feel about this service user and our work together? What does my reaction tell me about myself and about the case?'

Secondly, get to know yourself and your own psychological dynamics. Experiential learning and reflective practice may help you with this process. In *Chapter 2* you were introduced to techniques such as the Johari's window and illuminative incident analysis. You can use these to reflect on your own role in situations you encounter and to learn about yourself through your experiences in professional contexts. If you discover that there are unresolved issues from your past that hinder your professional effectiveness, you could seek counselling or psychotherapy to help you deal with these.

Thirdly, use your supervision effectively. Strong and potentially unhelpful reactions to service users need to be contained in supervision and potentially through seeking outside help, while reactions that help you understand the people you support better, need to be considered objectively to make sure that your work remains within the boundaries of good practice.

Fourthly, if you find that a particular group of service users routinely elicit unhelpful reactions in you, you might need to be a little selective in who you take on. You are less likely to be able to help someone who elicits a strong negative emotion in you, but you may also not be best placed to help someone who elicits a strong nurturing urge in you either. In both cases, use supervision to help you make good decisions and practise safely.

Fifthly, it is very important to be aware of your own motives – why you do the job you do. Sometimes people come into caring professions because they are searching for nurturance themselves. Do you need or want something from service users that they can't give you? If you think that this is the case, get the right kind of help for yourself, because you may still be excellently suited to your job, but you need the right kind of support so that you do not look to service users to meet your own emotional needs.

FOR THE JOURNAL

Think of a situation where you came across either a very strong reaction in yourself or in a service user in the course of your work. Choose a practice story or incident that illustrates the emotions concerned. In your journal, use one of the visual techniques presented in *Chapter 2*, such as illuminative incident analysis, to illustrate the incident you chose. Now work through the CLT reflective cycle to reflect on your experience. If you have learned anything about yourself during the course of this process, you can write it into a Johari's window framework. The extended example that follows on from this chapter contains an example of how to use some of these reflective techniques as an aid to understanding transference and countertransference reactions between practitioners and service users.

CHAPTER SUMMARY

Five key points to take away from Chapter 10:

- Strong feelings in both practitioners and service users are part and parcel of the work in frontline services.

- Some of these feelings may be displaced emotions from other key relationships in our lives.

- Transference refers to displaced emotions experienced by service users and directed towards practitioners. Countertransference operates in the opposite direction: These are displaced emotions from earlier (possibly unresolved) conflicts in the lives of practitioners. These feelings are felt towards service users.

- The strategies available to practitioners for dealing with service users' transference reactions include naming and talking about the reaction, working through the significance of the transference emotions in the individuals' lives, setting clear boundaries regarding limits and service expectations with the service user, and ensuring consistent practice across members of the team.

- Countertransference reactions can be so overwhelming or powerful that they prevent effective casework, but they can also be very useful tools to help practitioners understand what is happening in the lives of service users. The key to using countertransference reactions effectively is acknowledging these and developing personal awareness of the significance of these feelings to us. While actively pursuing enhanced self-awareness through reflective practice, practitioners can harness their countertransference feelings to understand service users better and to develop effective and innovative ways of working that acknowledge the complex emotions involved and foster containment. Making effective use of supervision to come to an understanding of countertransference reactions augments reflective work and ensures that practitioners are able to find containment themselves for these emotions.

FURTHER READING

There are two excellent sources that will help you to explore further the material covered in this chapter; namely, Lynette Hughes and Paul Pengelly's book *Staff Supervision in a Turbulent Environment* and Patrick Casement's book *On Learning from the Patient*.

SUGGESTED ANSWERS TO THE EXERCISE ON p. 137

There are no clear right or wrong answers. Supervision (option 6) is always helpful and should be sought almost without exception. The following responses are suggested by the author as being appropriate to the situations described under most circumstances where situations like the ones described in the vignettes occur in practice.

Vignette a): Person's reaction linked to their history; involvement of service is to support; it would be very helpful to come to a point where you can ask the question, 'I feel you are quite angry with me and the service, could it be because of the tough time you had in the past as a child in care, away from your parents? Or do you feel that it is something that I am doing now that is upsetting you?'

So, the suggested answer is 2.

Vignette b): Overly dependent service user. If you know the person very well, exploring the reasons behind their behaviour may be helpful for them to get to know themselves better. However, an effective response that does not require insight on the part of service users would be answers 3 and 4, which are about stating clearly what the boundaries of involvement are, and what expectations service users and the service have of one another. In this regard the idea of competence-promoting support, mentioned in *Chapter 6*, is also relevant.

Vignette c): Ashley is becoming overly dependent on the service and keeps asking for support that goes beyond the remit of the team. Appropriate response would be to clarify the limits and set up clear expectations of what can be provided with Ashley. It would also be appropriate to ensure the team treat Ashley with consistency (responses 3, 4 and 5).

Vignette d): The young person would benefit from reflecting on the impact of his past on his present behaviour. Due to the intensity and therapeutic nature of relationships between residential carers and the young people they work with, the first and second potential responses would be appropriate.

EXTENDED EXAMPLE 3

WORKING WITH CONTAINMENT AND TRANSFERENCE REACTIONS

Katy is a graduate mental health worker in a Child and Adolescent Mental Health (CAMHS) team who work with looked-after children. A few months ago Katy started to work with Jimmy, a three year old boy in foster care whose birth mother was a victim of people trafficking. She died from a drug overdose a few weeks after being freed from the gang who held her while awaiting repatriation. Jimmy's foster parents are a professional couple who asked for help with Jimmy's night terrors and support in getting him settled in a bedtime routine.

Katy first became aware of an unusual reaction in herself when, during visits to Jimmy's home, she started feeling irritated with the foster mother. Katy felt that she was looking down on her and dismissed advice as if she felt that she knew better. She felt herself increasingly drawn to the lively little boy, and then over the course of a weekend, she had the same dream on three nights in succession: she dreamt that she was kidnapped and kept tied up and blindfolded by a violent gang, followed by a dream scene where she gives birth to a baby boy. At that point in the dream she woke up on the first two nights. On the third occurrence of the dream, she saw the child's face – it was Jimmy.

After her recurring dream, Katy knew that her own reaction to the case needed some work. She spent some time reflecting on her role in the case and her reactions to Jimmy and the foster carer, and asked her supervisor for an extended supervision session on the case. The following extracts are drawn from her journal and from the conversation she had in supervision.

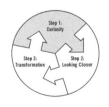

Katy's reflective cycle

Curiosity

These dreams really shook me. I've never had a reaction to anyone I worked with that was so strong that the case even featured in my dreams. The strange thing is that I was only aware of two emotions in my reaction to the case and I thought they were quite normal: I felt sorry for Jimmy. I think he went through a lot and he's such a lovely little boy. Could I have become too attached to him? I am not aware of spending more time with him than with anyone else in a similar situation in the past. My other emotion was irritation with the foster mum. She might be a professional in her own right, but I really felt she was out to put me down and very clear about my advice being rubbish. In fact, I guess the strongest feelings I was aware of while working with this family was after my last visit when I was very upset because she was very condescending and disrespectful towards me. I felt looked down on and almost punished, as if I was incompetent and had nothing to offer that would help Jimmy get better.

I wonder what my dreams could mean? Do they mean that in my unconscious I really want to be Jimmy's mother? Could there be another explanation; perhaps I am angry at the foster mum and this is my unconscious response. Have I got too close?

This is the first time in my career I have experienced this. Do my dreams mean I cannot work with this family any more? What will it feel like to do my next visit to their home?

How do I raise this in supervision without looking like I've already overstepped the boundaries? I know I need to talk about this with my supervisor, but I am very uncomfortable with the idea. What if I come across as really incompetent?

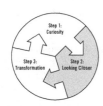

Looking closer

I am going to start with the easy questions. Supervision: I've always had lots of management supervision from my line manager and when it came to discussing cases, everything was mostly fine in the past. I tended to ask for advice on thorny issues that involved the management of cases. When I think about it, I am very frightened to take my emotions, and what might be my unconscious reactions to a case, to my supervisor – I've never done this before. So I guess my dreams have shown up a weakness in the way I've used supervision in the past. I've always felt it was really important to be confident and competent at your job. Feelings about my workload were OK too, as having too many things to do did not make you incompetent. But this really scares me. I could really look like I've become too involved with Jimmy and his foster mum. That makes me feel that I am not good enough or maybe that I should not do this kind of work. Maybe I am not cut out for it. I feel ashamed.

I think what I should do is just to take the bull by the horns. I'll tell my supervisor and see what happens, because if I don't, I won't be able to work effectively with Jimmy's case any more, and, anyway, maybe I'll learn something.

What do my dreams mean? Could they mean that I am over-involved? That I want Jimmy as my son? That I want to displace his foster mum? I simply don't know. But while I was feeling OK to work the case until I had the dreams, I think I have now become too upset. My feelings towards Jimmy and his foster mum don't relate to reality, so they are very possibly countertransference reactions. I don't like the sound of that, but it's probably the truth.

Are my feelings standing in the way of effective work?

When does countertransference get in the way of providing effective support? (see Chapter 10)

Table E3.1 *Katy's analysis of her countertransference feelings*

1. When these feelings are not recognised.	I think I've recognised a personal reaction to this case that could be a countertransference reaction.
2. When they become so strong, casework can no longer be effective.	I am very upset about my dreams, and that is why I need to get supervision. I am not sure if my dreams mean I can't work the case any more.
3. When you cannot do the work you are supposed to do, e.g. collusion to avoid an important issue.	I think this might be true, although I am not sure that I am unable to do the work. That's what I want to talk to my supervisor about.

Where do my feelings come from? It may be that I have a strong reaction to the case – I've always been upset by stories about people trafficking, drugs and suicide. There is no history of any of these things in my life and I grew up in a stable home – perhaps the origin of my feelings is just that I want Jimmy to have a stable home so much. But then I feel the same about all my cases and I don't get recurrent dreams about the other people I work with. I cannot figure it out.

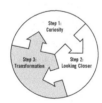

Transformation

What am I going to do about this? The first thing is to summarise what I've learned:

- I've become aware of a strong reaction in myself to a case and I cannot explain that reaction.

- Thinking through my reaction has lead me to learn some things about how I have used supervision in the past for safe discussions relating to case management and management issues rather than to talk about my feelings about cases.

- My reaction to the dreams has been very strong – I was very upset and that meant that I felt I needed to do some more work on my feelings through reflection and supervision.

- I learned some things about myself that I can note in my Johari's window:

Table E3.2 *Katy's Johari's window*

	Known to **others**	Unknown to **others**
Known to **self**	**Open** Happy to admit weaknesses to manager as long as these are OK to admit to, e.g. high workload.	**Hidden** Feelings of shame regarding my reaction to this case, in case I look incompetent and over-involved.
Unknown to **self**	**Blind** Avoidance in supervision of difficult case work & issues relating to emotions.	**Unknown** Recurrent dreams about a case that is upsetting. I think I might have had a countertransference reaction, but I am unaware of the emotional conflict it refers to or where the feelings are displaced from.

Katy went on to further reflect on the case in supervision. The following is an extract from the conversation with her supervisor:

Katy: I was worried about bringing this here. What if you thought I was really incompetent at my job and that I had got too involved with the family?

Supervisor: What do you feel now?

Katy: I feel better. You did not judge me and gave me good advice. I feel less ashamed of how I feel about Jimmy and all the other cases.

Supervisor: The other families? Do you have similar feelings about some of your other cases?

Katy: No, but I am not neutral towards everyone I work with and I was worried that to admit it would mean I am unprofessional.

Supervisor: What is different for you now?

Katy: I feel that it is OK to come here and say, I feel this way about so and so, even if it is a really strong or really negative feeling. It's like ... we can talk about it here and sort it out.

Supervisor: Without judgement?

Katy: Yes, I don't think you will judge me.

Supervisor: What about practising safely? That probably cuts both ways.

Katy: What do you mean?

Supervisor: Well, part of my role is to ensure that you practise safely. That means that children and families should get a good and responsible service, which in turn means that practitioners should practise to professional standards. But also that you, as a practitioner, feel safe in doing the work. That is, that we provide you with adequate support and guidance but also with protection and a safe space to talk when you feel overwhelmed like you just did. What are your thoughts on this?

Katy: I think that is right, and I feel OK about it, although today has been upsetting for me.

Supervisor: In particular?

Katy: Admitting that I must have felt very strongly drawn to Jimmy. That I felt a little like I did want to be his mum. You made that feel OK, that it wasn't a terrible thing ... to care. To really care.

Supervisor: It isn't a terrible thing, you know, to care about the people you work with.

Katy: I know, but I felt so ashamed about it. That I woke up feeling really frightened night after night after that dream.

Supervisor: And that might reflect an emotion from somewhere in the case?

Katy: Yes, I guess. Perhaps my dream gave me some of Jimmy's feelings about his mum. When she was being forced to do things she did not want to, or took drugs. It must've been very frightening for him. Maybe my night terrors were a little bit like his are.

Supervisor: We don't know that for sure, but it may be material you can learn from. I would like you to reflect some more on that for me. We still need to talk about how you will manage Jimmy's case from now on and also about how you are going to use supervision differently in future, but these last few minutes have been quite intense. Also for me. And very useful. Shall we take a five minute break and come back to finish our session?

Discussion questions

1. What are your thoughts on the reflective process that Katy went through? Do you think she used her journal and the CLT cycle effectively? How did that prepare her for talking about the case in supervision?
2. During the supervision dialogue, Katy had two insights that she had not thought about in her reflective journal. What were those? (The answers are: 1) That she also has strong feelings of caring about other cases which she was afraid of acknowledging in supervision; and 2) that her feelings of fear and terror during the dream could have

been a reflection of Jimmy's night terrors.) Can you think of a time when you had a completely new insight into a piece of work you were doing during a conversation in supervision, or while reflecting on the case with a colleague?

3. In light of the information given about Katy and Jimmy in this case study, what are your views on whether or not it is safe for Katy to continue working with Jimmy? Think about issues relating to boundaries (*Chapter 6*), ethics and values (*Chapter 8*), emotional containment (*Chapter 9*), and transference and countertransference (*Chapter 10*).

4. Look back at the dialogue between Katy and her supervisor. Using the concept of containment, as discussed in *Chapter 9*, how did the supervisor work with Katy to make it OK for her to give an honest account of her experience in supervision? (You can use the three-step containment process described in *Chapter 9* to structure your answer. The steps are: connect with the emotion, maintain an active presence, and facilitate closure.)

5. Can you name the areas of practice touched on in the dialogue where you feel Katy might work differently in future?

6. If someone in your team had a similar experience to Katy, how would it be dealt with? How far from ideal is that in your view? How can you go about fostering changes in the right direction?

PART FOUR

REFLECTING ON STAFF SUPPORT IN FRONTLINE SERVICES

11

ALL FOR ONE AND ONE FOR ALL: BUILDING SUPPORTIVE TEAMS

THIS CHAPTER AIMS TO:

- Help you reflect on what makes strong and effective teams;

- Challenge you to reflect on your own contribution to team work;

- Help you identify the team roles you take on in teams you are part of.

Frontline services are often organised in team structures. When teams work well, services are efficient and effective, and team members feel supported. Strong teams enhance resilience in the workplace and job satisfaction among practitioners. Dysfunctional teams, on the other hand, can be a source of frustration for team members and service users alike, and can exacerbate job stress and dissatisfaction at work.

REFLECTIVE ACTIVITY

If you are covering this chapter as part of a group, the following exercise might be a helpful ice-breaker to get the discussion started. If you are working through this book on your own, you can use the exercise for your journal.

Make a drawing or a diagram that shows your team at a typical team meeting. How do team members position themselves in the room? How does the communication typically flow? Who has a lot to say and who speaks very little? Does the amount people speak at team meetings reflect their status in the team? Do the people who speak a lot talk the most sense? When, where and by whom are the real decisions made? If you are very brave, you can try to depict each team member as a different animal and explain your reasons to the group. What can you infer about the functioning of your team from your drawing or diagram?

WHAT MAKES A TEAM STRONG?

As mentioned above, many frontline services are team-based. Teams provide members with reference groups for work-norms, social support, a sense of belonging, and a group of fellow practitioners to reflect and share ideas with. Supportive teams play an important role in helping to combat stress and burnout among staff. However, teams can also be dysfunctional and destructive. A destructive team dynamic can be very detrimental to team morale and have far-reaching effects, not only on the wellbeing and job satisfaction of individual team members, but also on the effectiveness of the team in delivering services.

The next two exercises invite you to explore both the positive and negative sides of team dynamics.

REFLECTIVE ACTIVITY

Think about a situation you are aware of where team working went wrong due to difficulties with the team dynamics. Through discussion and reflection see if you can answer the following questions about your example:

- What was the problem?

- Who was involved?

- Who was affected and how?

- What was the impact on team functioning?

- What was the impact on service delivery?

The following worked example might help you with the task.

Table 11.1 *The impact of negative team dynamics*

Problem	Who was involved?	Who was affected and how?	Impact on team functioning	Impact on service delivery
One team member frequently late for work or meetings asking others	Everyone in the team as everyone was asked to help out on many occasions.	All team members had a growing sense of frustration as it felt almost cruel to refuse to help out a colleague in	Reduced morale for everyone. Team was 'split' into two groups, an 'angry' group and a 'supportive'	Not immediate, but some team members noticed that they were becoming less willing to go the

Problem	Who was involved?	Who was affected and how?	Impact on team functioning	Impact on service delivery
to cover for her or 'rescue' her.		need; everyone's workload increased because one person did not pull their weight. This was a difficult issue to take to our manager as no one on the team wanted to get their colleagues in trouble.	group; many team members lost patience with their colleague who was not pulling her weight.	extra mile or to be as supportive to service users as before; some team members occasionally missed deadlines due to spending time 'helping out'.

This example shows that even relatively small issues can grow over time and eventually impact on service delivery. What did you notice about the impact of team dynamics on service delivery in the examples you came up with?

Team dynamics can be affected by many external and internal factors including management style, organisational change, interpersonal conflicts within the team, and the degree to which team members have a clear and congruent understanding of the role and purpose of the team, as we shall see in the next section.

REFLECTIVE ACTIVITY

Think back to a time when you were part of a strong team. It does not have to be a work team, but could be a sports team or any other team you were part of. What do you think were the characteristics of this team that made it strong? What was your role in the team in your example? How did this team deal with individual differences in strengths and weaknesses among the members? How was the team led?

Strong teams show the following nine characteristics (Payne, 2001):
1. A shared purpose or mission that is meaningful to members
2. Clear, measurable goals
3. A collaborative way of working together
4. Well-defined roles and responsibilities
5. Everyone shares in the accountability

6. A willingness to learn and develop the team's functioning
7. Participation in decision making and planning
8. Passion and enthusiasm
9. Celebrating work well done together.

When you think of the strong team in the previous exercise, how did it rate on these factors? What are the strengths or weaknesses for your team? Which areas need more attention? You can make a checklist for yourself where you rate your team functioning on a scale of 1 to 10 on these nine factors, as in the table below.

Table 11.2 *Team functioning checklist*

Indicator	Rating (0–10)	What we can do to improve
1. A shared purpose or mission that is meaningful		
2. Clear, measurable goals		
3. A collaborative way of working together		
4. Well-defined roles and responsibilities		
5. Everyone shares in the accountability		
6. A willingness to learn/develop the team's functioning		
7. Participation in decision making and planning		
8. Passion and enthusiasm		
9. Celebrating work well done together		

How can you address those areas you feel are weak for your team? Do you think your team would be able to take ownership of any of the identified areas that need improvement? Perhaps it might be helpful to take the checklist above to a team meeting and ask everyone for their perspective. Teams openly discussing difficulties can lead to straightforward solutions that really work because the whole team takes ownership of their plans (in contrast to imposed solutions that may not work within the practical constraints faced by the team).

INDIVIDUALS AND TEAM ROLES: WHERE DO I FIT IN?

Can you make a list of all the teams you belong to? You might be surprised how many there are, as work-based teams may not just encapsulate service lines or management relationships. You may be part of committees or work groups; perhaps you are part of teams outside the workplace. In all of these teams, you play a part and therefore have a contribution to make.

Have you noticed how people take on different roles within the teams they work in? Some individuals generate large numbers of creative ideas, while others are natural leaders who can help their teams to work in structured and efficient ways towards a goal when they are immersed in chaos; and other team members are able to focus their efforts on the hard work needed to complete the team's tasks.

People vary in the roles they take on within teams, and one person can have more than one role in any specific team, or play different roles in different teams they belong to over time. However, most of us tend to naturally take on a small number of specific roles in teams we form part of.

THE BELBIN* CLASSIFICATION OF TEAM ROLES

Do you find yourself drawn to take on specific roles in the teams you belong to? For example, do you regularly find that you are good at generating ideas for the team or do you find yourself becoming the coordinator or spokesperson for your team? Are you a 'grafter' or does your strength lie in delegating tasks to others? Industrial psychologist Meredith Belbin studied the phenomenon of team roles over many years and came up with a list of general team roles that capture the varied tasks that the vast majority of teams face in work environments.

The following table contains a list of the different team roles, their descriptions, and an 'allowable weakness' for each. Belbin believes that we can take on more than one of the team roles. We normally have a 'top three' of roles that we incline towards. We may also be able to take on some roles competently for short periods of time, including some least preferred roles. When you read through the list below, try to think which of these roles are your three preferred and three least preferred team roles and mark those in the boxes on the table.

> **REFLECTIVE ACTIVITY**
>
> 1. Can you think of recent examples where you took on one of your preferred roles in a team context? What about your least preferred roles?
>
> 2. Do the teams you are part of have members taking on all of these roles, or are there some roles that are absent or not needed?
>
> 3. When you think about the various team roles present in your work teams, are there some that are conspicuous by their absence? What do you think are the implications of this for the team's functioning?

*Belbin is a registered trade mark of Belbin Associates UK; Belbin materials adapted with kind permission from Belbin Associates UK.

Table 11.3 *Belbin team role descriptions*

Team role	Characteristic	Allowable weakness	Your preferred team roles	Your least preferred team roles
'Plant' (as in factory)	'Ideas factory' Creative, imaginative, unorthodox. Can solve difficult problems by thinking outside the box.	Ignores details. Can be too preoccupied with ideas to communicate effectively.		
Coordinator	Natural leader and chairperson. Confident and mature. Good delegator. Helps team to clarify goals and make good decisions.	Can be seen as manipulative or offloading own work onto others.		
Monitor/ Evaluator	Sees all the options, discerning. Can think strategically without getting overly emotional. Good judgement.	Can lose momentum and does not inspire others.		
Implementer	Diligent, disciplined and reliable and efficient; conservative; turns ideas into practical reality.	A little inflexible and slow to respond to new possibilities.		
Completer Finisher	Painstaking, conscientious, and precise; can be a good troubleshooter; will make sure the end result is perfect, but tends to be anxious.	Worries about the rules; does not delegate.		

Team role	Characteristic	Allowable weakness	Your preferred team roles	Your least preferred team roles
Resource Investigator	Explores new opportunities and develops new contacts; extrovert and enthusiastic and communicative.	Can be over-optimistic and also prone to lose enthusiasm fast if initial interest fades.		
Shaper	Challenging and dynamic with a rebellious edge; can be the 'devil's advocate'. Thrives on pressure and can overcome obstacles.	Can provoke and offend; speaks own mind, can lack tact.		
Teamworker	Cooperative, mild, perceptive and diplomatic. Listens well, averts friction.	Indecisive when pressure is high.		
Specialist	Self-starting; single-minded, dedicated. Has scarce knowledge.	Focused on technicalities and a narrow range of contribution.		

Adapted from material supplied by Belbin Associates; used with permission.
Team role descriptions: © Belbin Associates UK.

FOR THE JOURNAL

Spend some time reflecting on the roles you take on within the teams you are a part of. Record in your journal any observations you may have, especially about your own functioning in teams. How can you develop your practice so that you become an even stronger team member?

CHAPTER SUMMARY

Five key points to take away from Chapter 11:

- Many frontline services are organised around teams. Team working provides practitioners with many benefits including access to social support, a group with shared goals, and others to reflect and share ideas with.

- When team dynamics are affected by difficulties – even relatively small problems such as someone being habitually late for work – this can have a very detrimental impact on team functioning and team morale, affecting most if not all aspects of the team's functioning.

- Research into strong teams indicates that they share a number of characteristics including the following: a shared purpose, clear goals, collaborative working, well-defined roles, shared accountability, openness to learn and develop, participation in decision making, passion and enthusiasm, and celebrating work well done.

- Individuals within teams take on specific team roles which are functions that enable the team to complete its task effectively. Most teams need people to take on all nine of the team roles in order to function well, although one person can take on more than one role.

- The nine Belbin team roles are: Plant (person who generates ideas), Coordinator, Monitor/Evaluator, Implementer, Completer/Finisher, Resource Investigator (explores new opportunities), Shaper, Team Worker, and Specialist.

FURTHER READING

There is a huge literature on teams, team building and team functioning. Even a cursory search with any internet search engine should yield thousands of links to follow up. A good place to start if you would like to find out more about the Belbin team roles is Meredith Belbin's *Team Roles at Work,* second edition.

A website with some very helpful practical resources to help you develop your team is that of the Social Care Institute for Excellence, http://www.scie.org.uk/. Go to the resources section and look for the free downloads in the 'workforce development' section.

ACKNOWLEDGEMENT

Material on team roles used with the kind permission of Belbin Associates UK.

12

MAKING SENSE OF TANGLES, TWISTS AND TURNS: EFFECTIVE CASE SUPERVISION IN FRONTLINE PRACTICE

THIS CHAPTER AIMS TO:

- Define case supervision;

- Delineate the three functions of supervision;

- Explain what happens in supervision by distinguishing between different 'supervisory spaces';

- Apply the concept of the supervision triangle;

- Support practitioners to reflect on their development as reflective supervisees.

WHAT IS CASE SUPERVISION?

REFLECTIVE ACTIVITY

1. How would you define supervision?

2. Do you receive different kinds of supervision?

3. Who supervises you, how often, and for how long?

4. What happens in a typical supervision session?

Case supervision in the context of this chapter can be defined as follows:

Case supervision is a formal process within an organisation that involves overseeing and governing professional practice. Case supervision has one overarching aim, namely, to ensure high quality services. This is achieved through ensuring good quality and safe casework practice.

This definition points to the three essential elements for embedding good supervisory practice in frontline services. First, supervision should have a high priority within the organisation as a whole. Ensuring that all practitioners are provided with good quality supervision is not an optional extra, but an essential aspect of providing safe, high quality services.

The second important element in the definition of supervision is that the ultimate aim of supervision is the provision of high quality services to service users. Supervision is primarily about making sure that service users are well served, not about the supervisor or the supervisee's personal interests. However, good case supervision does involve practitioner development – the third element – as highly skilled and competent practitioners are more likely to deliver safe and high quality services.

At this point in the chapter, you may have noticed that we are talking about a very specific kind of supervision. There are, of course several types of supervision. The definition given above makes it clear that the kind of supervision considered in this chapter is 'clinical' or 'case' supervision, rather than operational or management supervision. A simple, yet helpful way to distinguish between the two kinds of supervision is to think of case supervision as directly concerning services provided to service users by the supervisee, while management or operational supervision is more concerned with human resources and management issues such as annual leave, appraisals of performance, and how resources are utilised.

There is a further dimension to understanding case supervision that is not explicitly mentioned in the definition above, and this is that supervision is usually provided by members of staff that are more experienced or senior to the supervisee. Although the reasons for this may seem obvious, it is still worth reflecting for a moment on why you think this is the case. In particular, does a good supervisor show competencies that are more than simply a higher level of technical mastery or more years of experience on the job? We explore the processes inherent in supervision below. As you work though these sections, try to remain alert to the competencies a good supervisor shows, as this may have implications for the quality of supervision you receive or, if you are a supervisor, give.

WHAT CAN SUPERVISION DO FOR ME? THE THREE FUNCTIONS OF CASE SUPERVISION

Case supervision serves a number of functions. Practitioners use supervision to find out what to do in particular situations, to talk through difficult moments they have encountered during the course of their work, or for identifying areas of practice that they may want to develop further.

A succinct way to capture these three functions of case supervision has been devised by Inskipp and Proctor (1993). They identified the following three functions of case supervision:

Formative: This aspect of supervision involves learning how to do the work. Formative supervision can range from being told what to do or how to accomplish a specific task, through to identifying a skills deficit that calls for further training.

Normative: Normative supervision involves support on aspects of practice where compliance with policies, procedures, guidelines or ethical codes is required. Normative supervision can take the form of clear guidance, or of a facilitated process of ethical decision making.

Restorative: Restorative supervision provides a containing space for practitioner emotions. In this sense supervision parallels therapy. Restorative supervision involves exploring how things are for practitioners. Restorative supervision supports the emotional impact on practitioners of working in frontline services. Strong emotions are normalised and the implications and learning from transference and countertransference reactions are worked through. The duty of care of the organisation towards members of staff whose wellbeing is put at risk by the emotional impact of their work on them forms a legitimate focus of restorative supervision, inasmuch as supervisors have a duty to encourage practitioners to develop effective ways to care for themselves.

REFLECTIVE ACTIVITY

Supervisors are usually senior or more experienced members of staff than those they supervise. Consider the formative, normative and restorative functions of supervision described above. How would seniority or additional experience of the supervisor contribute to the quality of supervision provided to practitioners? Can you distinguish between the contributions of seniority (in rank), the value of additional work-related experience, and more general life experience in the quality of supervision in your answers above?

Consider the following case study:

> You strongly suspect that Kirsty, a young mother you are working with, has become clinically depressed during the last few weeks. She is much less motivated and cooperative than she had been previously. You are also concerned about the welfare of her children. While you discuss her case with your supervisor, you suddenly remember a time, many years ago, when you felt very depressed yourself.

Consider the three functions of supervision outlined above and answer the following questions:

1. Which personal or professional dilemmas would Kirsty's case raise for you? What do you need from your supervisor in terms of the restorative component of supervision?

2. How do you think a supervisor with more life or work experience might respond differently to you, given your own history of depression?

3. What would you expect from the formative and normative aspects of supervision in such a case?

UNDERSTANDING THE PROCESS OF CASE SUPERVISION: SUPERVISORY SPACES

There are a number of different ways in which case supervision can be helpful in supporting frontline practice. All of these underpin the normative, formative and restorative components of supervision.

Supervision as narrative space

Case supervision provides the space where a number of different narratives intersect. The narratives of service users as related by practitioners meet the narratives of the agency, the supervisee, and also that of the supervisor. These stories and their mutual influence unfold within the case work. In the chapter on narrative approaches, we considered the power of enabling service users to re-author their own stories. Supervision is the place where practitioners and services set the parameters within which such potential re-authoring takes place.

Viewing supervision as a form of mutual storytelling brings to the fore the powerful influence of labelling exerted in case work; how people are represented within supervision can have a significant effect on the eventual responses of agencies that provide services. Depending on how supervisees present the 'story' of cases, supervisors may respond in different ways. The following reflective activity illustrates this point:

REFLECTIVE ACTIVITY

Think of a recent case that you took to supervision and how you told your supervisor about the service user. How did your supervisor react to the services user's narrative as told by you? Were there any aspects of your supervisor's reaction that may have been influenced by how you presented the case?

For instance, how did you start talking about the case with your supervisor? What did your first sentence and your body language say about how you view the people you talked about? Was your account coherent, complete and filled with narrative depth, or was it unstructured, full of omissions, and lacking due consideration of the complexities of the different characters in the 'plot'? How does the way you narrated your case reflect what was happening for the service user and what was happening for you? What was your supervisor's response to the story you told?

If you found examples of how the way in which you present cases affects the quality or content of the supervision you receive, can you think of ways that changing how you present your cases to your supervisor might help improve the quality of the supervision you receive?

The reflective activity above illustrates that many nuances implicit in the way you present your account of cases can affect the content and process of supervision. The narrative you construct in case supervision can be a reflection of the dynamics experienced by the service users you are talking about. The way the story you present is interpreted can affect the content of the supervision you receive. In turn, this can have a dramatic impact on your further management of the case, thereby affecting the experience of service users and, in turn, influencing future narratives on the part of service users, practitioners and supervisors in a continuous cycle. Breaking out of unhelpful self-perpetuating cycles really depends on practitioners and their supervisors cultivating self-awareness and personal reflection. Developing their own reflective practice in these ways will enable them to be alert to destructive processes in supervision and service delivery, enable them to challenge themselves or each other effectively, and take prompt remedial action where necessary.

Apart from the supervisor–supervisee dimension, there are also organisational and cultural narratives that may be active in the background of your work. For example, how does your organisation view the users of its services? Examples of different perspectives include constructing service users as helpless, infantile, ill or useless.

REFLECTIVE ACTIVITY

Within your organisation or your team, which narratives are prevalent about the users of your services? Do any of the following apply? Service users could be viewed as:

- Helpless, in need of support

- Clueless, in need of being told 'what is what'

- Child-like, in need of parenting

- Ill and in need of treatment

- Scroungers, who should be caught out/curtailed

- The 'deserving' poor

- The 'undeserving' poor

- Victims of society who should be protected from exploitation

- Perpetrators from whom society should be protected

- People in distress and chaos, in need of rescuing

If any of these apply, how does that affect the way services are provided and the ways in which staff talk about the people they work with?

Can you think of a recent case where one or more of these narratives were prevalent within your supervision? How did this affect the decisions or advice that you took from the supervision session? How would things have been different if the narrative was reversed; for example, instead of thinking about service users as helpless and incapable, they were viewed with assumptions of competence and cooperation? Did you notice any self-fulfilling prophecies or unhelpful self-perpetuating cycles?

Can you identify narratives or discourses within your service about service users that are muted or suppressed? A clue would be to think of what is currently defined as 'politically incorrect' language to use – especially in instances where there are sizeable numbers of people who hold a view but may be afraid to express it. Alternatively, you might be aware of opinions that are prevalent among staff but that they would be very reluctant to express in public. Many examples of this phenomenon are controversial; for instance discourses on asylum seekers, immigration, gender bias, racism, and politics are often (rightly) muted within the workplace. However, these issues are present in people's minds and can exert an influence on how services are provided to individuals that is not openly acknowledged by either the organisation or individual practitioners or their supervisors.

If you are aware of such muted discourses, what is the impact of these on the way services are provided? What would be the advantages and disadvantages of more openly talking about the issues involved? How can you bring this issue into your own case supervision?

REFLECTIVE ACTIVITY

Take a well-known fairy tale, change some of the characters around, and retell it in such a way that it brings to the fore the way your service typically works with service users, the prevalent and muted discourses that operate in your service, and the social or political context within which you operate. For example, you could retell the story of Cinderella, casting her as an immigrant or asylum seeker, and turn the character of the fairy godmother into her social worker, and so forth. (See also the reflective activity on p. 29 (*Fig. 2.3*))

Supervision as a space to think

Part of the narrative that is constructed during case supervision consists of making sense of what is happening in the work with service users. Thinking through what is happening, problem solving, case conceptualisation, and resolving ethical and other professional dilemmas all need the safety and boundaries of supervisory space to happen effectively. Such thinking space within supervision is about rationality and responding professionally to situations that are inherently complex, where information is incomplete, and where emotions are highly charged.

To be able to think effectively, thinking space has to be available and free from unnecessary interruptions, and it also has to offer the opportunity for a special kind of silence that allows clear thinking to occur. This is why good supervisory practice respects the sanctity of supervision sessions and prioritises these above almost every other commitment.

Good supervisors do not tolerate interruptions either of the physical continuity of supervision sessions, or unnecessary intrusions into the mental processes of the supervisee.

Silence in this context refers to a mental quietness that allows practitioners the possibility to become absorbed in their thoughts about a case, to be alone, thinking, whilst in the presence of the supervisor (this is much like Winnicott's (1990) idea of infants learning to be alone in the presence of an 'other', i.e. their mother, before they develop the capacity to be truly by themselves). Following through on the analogy with infants' development of the capacity to be alone and learning to develop sound internalised thinking processes, good supervisory practice involves supervisors staying with the practitioner's process rather than imposing their own solutions to supervisee problems prematurely. A process of carefully guided discovery is more likely to facilitate mature thinking in practitioners than imposed solutions – even if the latter are 'correct'. Good supervisors purposely develop the skill of honing the extent to which they offer concrete advice and solutions to their supervisees (Casement, 1985; Winnicott, 2005).

Supervision as a space for enactment and containment

It is unavoidable that the emotions that accompany frontline practice are brought into the supervisory space. The narratives that supervisees present are bound to reflect the level of need and degree of distress experienced by service users. Practitioner feelings about the work, as well as feelings about service users, their own and other organisations, and vulnerabilities stemming from their own personal histories can all intrude into the discussion. Supervision therefore becomes the appropriate space for supervisees to make sense of the whole of what is happening for them.

Supervisors, in their responses to their supervisees, model the way in which mature practitioners within the organisation respond to the dynamics they encounter. For example, bringing to supervision a service user's disclosure that she is seriously considering suicide may set off a measured reaction from a supervisor that focuses on rational risk assessment leading to reasoned action. If, on the other hand, a supervisor responds with panic, the resulting service response may mirror the uncontained distress of the service user in question, and equally fail to contain practitioner emotions which may include anxiety, panic and an inflated sense of personal responsibility. Another example of how supervisors can facilitate mature practice through their own behaviour occurs when they make available in supervision a space where practitioners can openly work through mistakes and errors in judgement. Once again, supervisors responding with either blame or defensive manoeuvres model a culture of 'covering my own back' and opacity – the opposite of the openness and transparency that the public expect from services.

In summary, supervision as a space for containment involves providing for practitioners a safe space where they feel supported and encouraged to think and feel, where their own and others' strong feelings can be discussed openly and where sense-making occurs.

Supervision as a space for enactment of emotions links to the containment function. When practitioners' emotional reactions mirror the dynamics present in a case or when a work-related incident brings out deep personal anxieties in practitioners, the supervisory space offers permission to enact and experience these emotions, secure in the knowledge that supervisors will facilitate and contain their feelings and steer them along safe passages through the feelings that might be overwhelming. Although practitioners may experience emotions that reflect their own anxieties or present countertransference reactions to their clients (see *Chapter 10*), they may also bring to supervision emotions that are realistic responses to the experiences of service users. The task of the supervisor is to support enactment of these feelings in such a way as to facilitate the ability of supervisees to tell the difference. For instance, practitioners may experience legitimate sadness in reaction to a loss in the life of one of their clients. Alternatively, the reaction may be a displaced (countertransference) reaction stemming from a similar loss in the practitioner's life. Supervision can serve as a safe space where supervisees can experience strong emotions safely and then think through their reactions, devising thoughtful and appropriate ways of responding to service users.

Can you think of an example from your experience where case supervision has supported you in the ways discussed above? How did the supervisor support you in containing and enacting your own emotions?

If you cannot think of an actual example from your experience, try to think of a situation where this function of supervision would have been helpful. What, in supervision, would have helped you deal with the situation?

This enactment and containment function of supervision is the one element of supervisory practice that arguably overlaps most strongly with reflective practice. Do you think that reflective practitioners would respond differently to the exploration of their own emotions within supervision? If so, how would good supervisory practice be enhanced when supervisees are reflective in their approach to their work?

FOCUS ON THE SUPERVISION CONVERSATION: SUPERVISION TRIANGLES

How can our understanding of the supervisory process influence the content and process of actual supervision sessions? Is there a way we can map or measure what happens in supervision on a case by case or session by session basis so that our understanding of supervision 'theory' affects what we actually talk about? Hughes and Pengelly (1997) offer one such framework that is both conceptually simple and useful in practice. They pose the idea of a supervision triangle which considers every supervision discussion to involve three participants, even though one participant is not present in the room: the supervisor, supervisee, and the service user.

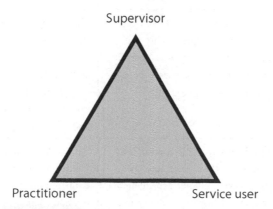

Figure 12.1 *The supervision triangle*
(From Hughes, L. & Pengelly, P. Staff supervision in a turbulent environment, *Fig. 3.1, p. 41. Reproduced by permission of Jessica Kingsley Publishers.)*

The focus of the conversation in case supervision has to cover all three corners of the triangle. Supervisors are tasked with providing guidance and support (normative, restorative and formative functions of supervision) to the supervisee. Supervisees, in turn, are tasked with narrating the story of service users in such a way that they can use the supervisory space effectively.

During the supervision conversation, each of the participants should get a turn to have their voices heard (even if not physically present in the room). There should be a degree of balance between the different perspectives explored, although equal time may not be ideal in all situations (Hughes & Pengelly, 1997). When there is a consistent imbalance – over- or underemphasis – of any of the three corners of the supervision triangle, the process becomes skewed, as illustrated in the following exercise.

REFLECTIVE ACTIVITY

Part 1

You are working with someone who has been really difficult to deal with in the last week and you take it to your supervision. Taking the three sides of the supervision triangle in turn, what do you think are examples of how imbalance in any one of those three elements can skew the supervision process?

Add your own thoughts to the table below:

Table 12.1 *Balancing the supervision conversation*

	Overemphasis	Underemphasis
Supervisor	Supervisor spends too much time talking about their own reaction to cases – does not listen to supervisee.	Leaves supervisee to figure it all out for themselves. Does not guide, give guidelines, or facilitate discovery or reflection.
Supervisee	Everything is framed as linked to the supervisee's personality or dynamics. 'It's all in how you handle it'; or supervision becomes a therapy session/counselling.	The management of the case or supervisee's own reaction to the work are not discussed, because other things are focused on, e.g. distraction into diagnosing and discussing the service user, or talking about other agencies and their failings in the case.
Service users	The problems are all located in the service user – they are seen as the 'sick' ones who will need to change their ways, without an appreciation of relevant contextual factors.	Service users are seen as helpless victims of circumstance and their contributions to their situations are not considered.

Part 2

For the journal

The journalling exercise for this chapter is to analyse your own supervision along the lines of this exercise. Take a decent sample of different cases you work with, say three to five different cases, and see if you can map out how the case discussions in supervision develop across the three sides of the supervision triangle. What did you learn from doing this exercise that might help you have more effective supervision experiences in future?

THE REFLECTIVE SUPERVISEE: DEVELOPING IN SUPERVISION

This final section briefly covers the process dimension of supervision over time. As practitioners become more confident and competent, they develop in their practice and also in what they need from case supervision. There are a number of developmental models that explore the ways in which supervisees gradually find their own voices within supervision (Milne, 2009; Scaife, 2001). The following description of this process draws on the author's own experience and on adult learning theory (Horwath & Morrison, 1999).

Imitation

As new trainees or students, practitioners very often feel overwhelmed by the complexities of the people they work with. They also tend to feel underprepared to deliver services in practice. Not infrequently, this is at the level of feeling totally incompetent. Supervisors are viewed as those in the know. They are admired for their knowledge, skill and experience, and any advice or guidance is followed closely and the supervisor's way of working is imitated as far as possible – often without question. Trainee practitioners at this stage may occasionally have views of their own, but these are very quickly subordinated to those of their supervisors.

Substitution

As learners develop, they become increasingly aware of their own emerging opinions and views. In frontline services in health and social care there are frequently no immediate right or wrong answers to difficult dilemmas, so experience, wisdom, opinion and technical knowledge all contribute to decision making. As trainee practitioners develop their own views, they may occasionally find themselves holding views that conflict with those of their supervisors, but these are fairly speedily and comprehensively replaced with those advocated by the supervisor as, after all, the 'supervisor knows best'.

Over time this phase continues, but learners may come to hold stronger views and become more confident in expressing these as they gain more experience and see for themselves how the guidance and advice they are given pans out. In practice, though, own views tend to be ignored and supervisor directives are still followed. However, practitioners become more aware of their own thinking and may occasionally covertly disagree with their supervisors. Their own views are, however, muted in favour of the supervisor's discourse.

Suppression

The next stage involves trainees finding themselves developing strong ideas of their own and the ability to disagree openly with their supervisors. They are able to defend their views, question received wisdom and debate various courses of action in supervision. They may also develop the ability to integrate the views of the supervisor with their own, without completely rejecting one set of ideas for another. They now become confident enough to follow their own courses of action on occasion – even if these are in conflict with those suggested to them in supervision. Overall, however, the supervisor's discourse is still privileged and their own views suppressed, but they do not allow the supervisor's views to replace or completely override their own opinions.

Integration

The final stage occurs when practitioners start asserting their own views in mature ways. They are able to reconcile potentially conflicting views without sacrificing their own ideas or actions in favour of those of the supervisor. They are able to use supervision for their restorative and normative needs, but require less formative input on their casework. They ask for and take on less concrete advice, and their own personalities and views become more visible in their approaches to their work.

This may also mean that courses of action are decided on autonomously and they develop an inner supervisory voice that provides them with guidance. The inner supervisory voice here is much the same concept as Casement's (1985) notion of an internal supervisor. Since practitioners themselves make the final decisions regarding the courses of action they take at this stage, they generally feel confident enough to go with their own opinions if they feel that these are more accurate or apt for the situation than those of the supervisor.

REFLECTIVE ACTIVITY

Where in this process do you see yourself? What are the challenges in your own development as a practitioner that you would like to address in your own supervision at this stage of your development?

The supervisor's role in supervisee development

Of course, for practitioners to develop to the level where they can openly disagree with supervisors and follow their own minds in cases of conflicting views, supervisors need to be open to their supervisees disagreeing with them and questioning their views. For some supervisors this can be an extremely difficult challenge in their own development. The normative function of supervision also requires that supervisors guard the limits of safe practice. Supervisee development is therefore fostered along the two dimensions of increasing confidence and competence on the one hand, and correspondingly, increasing levels of supervisor trust and openness in the supervisee–supervisor relationship on the other. Good supervisors are happy to be wrong sometimes or to have their supervisees experiment and learn from experience within appropriate limits which they, of course, enforce as part of their supervisory function.

REFLECTIVE ACTIVITY

Discuss the aforementioned phases of development in the supervisor–supervisee relationship with colleagues in your team.

1. What are your views on the stages mentioned? Do you agree or disagree with the idea that practitioners progress through these stages as they develop their practice?

2. What are the benefits and the risks that are raised in each of the phases? For instance, what are the risks for supervisees who follow supervisor directives without question? When you answer this question, try to consider the formative, normative and restorative functions of supervision. For instance, supervisees who never question supervisor guidance may not learn the reasoning processes that support decision making in their fields of practice (normative function).

3. How would these phases be affected by the journey towards becoming a reflective practitioner? Do you see differences or parallels in the process of becoming more reflective?

CHAPTER SUMMARY

Five key points to take away from Chapter 12:

↪ Case supervision is a formal process within organisations that oversees and governs professional practice. Its overarching aim is to ensure high quality services, delivered safely.

⊷ In practice, case supervision has three important facets: formative, normative and restorative. Formative elements of case supervision involve learning how to do the work; normative aspects are about keeping in step with standards, policies or guidelines; while restorative supervision revolves around helping practitioners deal with their own processes and emotions which might have surfaced during the course of their casework.

⊷ Case supervision can also be conceptualised as a set of spaces which provides the time and place for practitioners to reflect. In this chapter distinctions were drawn between supervision as narrative space (where the stories of services, practitioners, and service users intersect), supervision as a space to think, and supervision as a space for enactment and containment.

⊷ Effective supervisory conversations in this context involve achieving a balance between focusing on the service user, supervisee, and supervisor. Imbalances between these three elements can cause biased approaches to service users that that may be ineffective and unhelpful.

⊷ Supervisees develop their clinical skills over time. The developmental process frequently takes place in stages, starting with accepting all input from the supervisor without question (imitation), moving on to developing viewpoints of one's own but still substituting supervisors' ideas for one's own, and then developing to a point where supervisees increasingly suppress their own ideas in practice, while still holding on to them. Finally, supervisees might reach a stage of integration where they can hold different, even conflicting perspectives in mind and implement the most sensible course of action based on understanding all the relevant perspectives.

FURTHER READING

There are many good texts on supervision available. One of the most interesting and useful is that by Lynette Hughes and Paul Pengelly (1997) which was referred to frequently in the text of this chapter. For a very comprehensive summary of the various supervision models, the texts by Scaife (2001) and Milne (2009) in the references are both very helpful. Finally, if you would like to explore the psychodynamic concepts of containment in supervision and the internal supervisor, Patrick Casement's book, *On Learning from the Patient* is a good starting point, as is *Chapter 9* on emotional containment in this book.

13

WHEN THE GOING GETS TOUGH: STRESS AND BURNOUT IN FRONTLINE SERVICES

CHAPTER AIMS:

In this chapter you will learn:

- How to define stress;

- How people respond to stress;

- How to identify some early signs of chronic stress;

- The impact of stress on psychological functioning and physical wellbeing;

- How poorly-managed stress leads to burnout;

- How to manage and prevent unnecessary stress and burnout in individuals, teams and organisations;

- The role of reflective practice in dealing with staff stress.

THE STRESS RESPONSE

Throughout this book we have mentioned the emotional cost to practitioners of being constantly confronted with human need. Faced on a daily basis with people who are distressed through poverty, homelessness, trauma and mental or physical health problems can be an overpowering experience for staff in frontline services. Team members may also be faced with ethical dilemmas or situations where the constraints imposed by the very system they work in offend their sense of natural justice. Where such situations occur on a regular basis, practitioners may start to feel that their roles demand more from them than they are able to give. High levels of job stress can become commonplace, which is illustrated by the generally accepted statistic that sickness absence among staff in frontline services, especially in the public sector, is relatively high compared to other sectors of the economy (Health and Safety Executive, 2004).

What is stress?

Stress has become a ubiquitous term in industrialised societies. The word has been so overused in recent years that it has lost much of its meaning – nowadays just about anything can be viewed as a source of stress (Leher, Woolfolk & Sime, 2007). Yet stress related to work is a very serious problem. Statistics from the Health and Safety Executive (HSE) in the UK show that job stress costs the UK economy approximately £3.8 billion per year and causes an annual loss of 13.5 million working days (Health and Safety Executive, 1999).

REFLECTIVE ACTIVITY

How would you define stress? Would you say that all stress is bad for you? Can you think of examples where the term has lost most of its meaning? If so, what are the consequences of this for the workplace?

One way to conceptualise harmful stress sensibly is to consider stress to arise when individuals feel unable to meet the demands they face. This definition of stress alludes to two important components of stress. First of all, feeling stressed is a personal reaction – different individuals may experience different situations as stressful. Your appraisal of any situation will determine whether or not *you* feel under stress in that situation. Someone else may not. Generally, people tend to appraise those situations as stressful where they perceive they do not have the capacity or resources to cope (Bishop, 1994).

Secondly, we experience stress in interaction with our environments. The situations that might cause a nurse in a busy Accident and Emergency Unit to feel stressed are likely to be very different from the sources of stress for a social worker in a child protection team. Managing or preventing harmful stress in different kinds of organisations will consequently require different strategies. We will look at how to manage or prevent stress from an organisational perspective in a later section of this chapter.

How we respond to stress

When we are faced with situations where we experience the demands on us as exceeding our capacity to cope, the human stress response is triggered. At a physiological level, the stress response involves a part of the nervous system called the autonomic nervous system. The function of the autonomic nervous system is to regulate internal body organs. The physiological stress response is really nothing other than the well-known mechanism of 'fight, flight or freeze'. The box below explains in more detail how the two complementary parts of the autonomic nervous system work together with the endocrine (hormonal) system to prepare the body for its response to the stressful situation and, once the stress is over, to restore the body's balance and recover (Bishop, 1994).

How the endocrine and autonomic nervous systems manage the body's response to stress

The autonomic nervous system consists of two sets of nerve fibres called the sympathetic and parasympathetic nervous systems. Together these two neural pathways control how the internal organs operate. Examples of functions controlled by the autonomic nervous system include regulating the heart rate, breathing and digestion.

When the stress response is triggered, the sympathetic nervous system prepares the body physiologically to respond. Signals from sympathetic nerve fibres trigger the release of adrenaline and noradrenaline (two hormones) by the adrenal glands which are located at the top of the kidneys. These hormones work together with the sympathetic nervous system to increase cardiovascular activity, respiration and perspiration, muscle strength, and mental activity. Other sympathetic pathways stimulate the release of glucose by the liver to give the body the energy it needs to deal with the situation at hand. The pupils of the eyes are dilated, digestion slowed down, heartbeat speeded up, and the bladder relaxed. All of these actions are designed to free up the body's resources to deal with the threat. Apart from the hormones already mentioned, hormones from the pituitary gland in the hypothalamus (which is a part of the brain stem) work with the sympathetic nervous system to release hormones that increase energy release (blood glucose levels), and suppress the immune system. At the same time some of these stress hormones help suppress any inflammation or infection that might result from the body's attempts to deal with the threat it faces.

Once the individual perceives that the threat has subsided, the parasympathetic nervous system starts to counteract the changes brought about by the sympathetic nervous system. This enables the body to recover from the strain experienced on its resources and energy stores during the time when it dealt with the perceived threat. Parasympathetic activation slows down the heartbeat, stimulates digestion, and has a generally calming effect. In effect, parasympathetic activation is designed to bring the body back to normal.

Over time our bodies develop a balance between these two systems, with the parasympathetic system restoring equilibrium after the sympathetic nervous system primes the body for responding to threat. If the threats we face are constantly present, this balance ends up being skewed in the direction of high levels of autonomic arousal, as the body does not have time to recover fully between threats. As described above, the stress response also suppresses immune functioning. This partly explains why long-term exposure to high levels of stress can lead to people becoming more vulnerable to infections. We are victims of our own physiology as far as stress is concerned; the same response that our ancestors might have had to a hungry-looking sabre-toothed tiger now kicks in when we are faced with situations we perceive as threats at work. In other words, our bodies respond to psychological dangers in our environment using the same physiological systems that evolved to allow us to cope with physical dangers.

REFLECTIVE ACTIVITY

All of us face occasional stressful situations at work. How will you know that your level of work stress has moved beyond this to the level of chronic stress? There are a number of early signs that the balance mentioned above has shifted in an unhealthy direction. How many of the following statements are true for you?

1. I find it hard to switch off from work while away from the office or when on holiday.

2. I have difficulty sleeping, due to worrying about work-related issues.

3. I have been more irritable than usual lately.

4. I dread going in to work on most days.

5. I am finding it very hard to make decisions.

6. I have been off sick more than usual in the last few months.

7. I find myself working longer hours, but achieving less.

8. I have recently had incidents at work where I behaved out of character, for instance losing my temper with a client, subordinate or co-worker.

9. I have been drinking more than usual in the last few months.

10. I have been experiencing more frequent physical symptoms than usual; for example, frequent headaches or abdominal pain.

If you answered 'yes' to the majority of these statements, the chances are that you are experiencing high levels of work-related stress. Your employer may be able to help you address the issues that have caused you to feel under stress. In a later section of this chapter we consider what some of those mechanisms might be, but in the first instance talking to your line manager is usually a good place to start.

THE IMPACT OF STRESS

Many research studies have found links between stress and mental or physical ill-health (Bishop, 1994). Specifically, stressful life events and daily hassles – both work and non-work related – have been linked with psychological and physical symptoms. Some of the risks that are associated with chronic stress include high blood pressure, heart disease, and psychological conditions such as depression and anxiety disorders.

BURNOUT

Over the last few decades, research has shown that people doing certain kinds of work are prone to a specific form of work-related stress that has been called the burnout syndrome. Particularly vulnerable are nurses, doctors, social workers, teachers, people managers and staff in caring professions (Maslach, 1982). As you may have noticed from this list, a number of frontline services are included. Other practitioners who work in frontline services are also likely to be at risk of burnout to the extent that their work roles share the features we used earlier to define frontline services, namely the high level of emotional demand on staff, and daily exposure to other people's physical, psychological and social needs or distress.

REFLECTIVE ACTIVITY

Have you come across anyone you felt suffered from the burnout syndrome? How would you describe the symptoms they experienced? What was the impact on areas such as their work functioning, personal life and their team? How were these difficulties managed within the organisation? Can you think of any ways in which this could have been improved? Finally, if you were ever to find yourself in a position where you were close to burnout, how would you like the situation to be dealt with by work? Try to think of what you would expect from colleagues, your manager, and from your employing organisation.

Symptoms of burnout

People who suffer from burnout have been shown to experience the following symptoms:

Fatigue and depression

Emotional exhaustion, fatigue and depression are consistently rated as the most prevalent common features in burnout research. The person who is burnt out feels drained and tired. It is very difficult to face a day's work. Their perceptions are that they have given all they could and there is nothing left to offer.

Diminished sense of personal accomplishment and loss of confidence

All effort appears to be wasted and it feels as if nothing useful is achieved at work. Burnt out individuals question their own abilities and may feel they have lost their touch. They seriously question their own ability to do the job.

Depersonalisation

Staff who are burnt out feel distant and detached from others and disconnected from their job roles, and they may feel that they have stopped caring. A lack of enthusiasm and passion for the work becomes evident as burnout becomes more pronounced.

REFLECTIVE ACTIVITY

If you felt that most or almost all of the statements in the self-assessment for chronic stress were true for you, you may also be able to relate to some of the following:

1. I almost always find myself with insufficient time to do things at work I actually enjoy

2. I feel overwhelmed by the demands of my role

3. I find it very difficult to get to sleep for worrying about work-related issues

4. I feel as if I am starting to lose control at work. For example, I am very indecisive and I do not see things in their proper perspective

5. It feels as though I am just going through the motions

6. I am starting to feel my job is not worth while

7. I don't really make a difference to anyone in my job

8. I have stopped caring, I've lost my passion and enthusiasm

9. I am very prone to use procrastination as an avoidance strategy at work

10. I panic or feel a strong sense of dread about going in to work.

Although some of the questions in this list are similar to the signs of chronic stress mentioned earlier in this chapter, burnout can be seen as a more extreme outcome of chronic stress. If you feel that you might be suffering from burnout, you need to act now. Talk to your line manager or take some of the steps mentioned in the section on dealing with burnout, below.

How burnout develops

All of us, when placed under a high enough level of strain, can develop burnout. However, Maslach (1982) believes that certain kinds of individuals are somewhat more prone to burnout than others. She specifically mentions individuals with the following traits as being at increased risk:

- People with strong need for approval from others and the need to achieve at work;

- Individuals who are unassertive with others;

- People who strongly need to feel in control or on top of things.

However, she is also clear that everyone has a limit to the stress levels they can manage, and that therefore all of us are at some risk of burning out.

Individuals prone to burnout tend to respond to job demands and feelings of not being in control by working harder. Despite the extra effort, they may become less effective at work, feel emotionally drained, and become less able to make decisions or take appropriate perspectives on the problems they encounter at work. Feeling more out of control, they may respond by working even harder. They may deny difficulties at work even if these clearly affect their lives outside work. This means that, as their stress levels rise, they use their social support networks less effectively.

Three very important early warning signals for burnout are: becoming increasingly unable to stop thinking about work when at home, inability to make decisions, and giving up hobbies and friends because of feeling too tired or busy.

As burnout sets in, some individuals start avoiding those activities at work that could lead to peer or management support, such as team meetings and supervision. They may have frequent absences related to minor illnesses and going to work increasingly becomes a dreaded chore. Lapses of judgement start showing and performance at work deteriorates noticeably, despite the quantity of work put in. Managers sometimes pick up on some of the early signs, but they can be reluctant to challenge a member of staff who is known for their hard work and commitment. If their personal relationships deteriorate, the person burning out might start using work as a coping mechanism.

As the symptoms of full-blown burnout set in, work performance deteriorates further, lapses in judgement become more apparent, sickness absences increase, and the core symptoms of burnout (emotional exhaustion, depersonalisation and a diminished sense of personal accomplishment) become very apparent. At this stage, burnout is not infrequently accompanied by mental health problems such as clinical depression or an anxiety disorder.

Managing burnout

Burnt-out individuals often realise that they are simply not able to go in to work. Extended periods of stress-related sickness absence may result. Once someone is suffering from burnout, it is imperative that they receive help.

Maslach (1982) recommends a range of measures that can be taken to help someone who is experiencing burnout. A key recommendation is to ensure that the person accesses plenty of helpful social support – both from colleagues and from professional helpers if needed. Peer group support, restructuring workloads to ensure enough rest breaks, and sharing the emotional load of the work with others can all be helpful.

More in-depth help may also be needed. First of all, medication and professional therapy might be useful to address symptoms of anxiety and depression. Secondly, the affected individual may need to take an extended leave of absence from work to recover, gain a fresh perspective, and if they decide to return to work, they may need to do so with a managed or phased return. A key to recovery is re-visioning of one's own identity and finding new sources of vitality which might include undertaking a new challenge in the workplace or perhaps even a radical step such as changing careers.

HOW TO PREVENT UNNECESSARY STRESS AND BURNOUT IN INDIVIDUALS, TEAMS AND ORGANISATIONS

Organisations can do much to manage staff stress and prevent unnecessary stress and burnout among their employees. Usually organisational stress management takes place at three levels (Bamber, 2006). Primary prevention involves the way organisations design jobs, manage people through formal or informal structures, and create organisational cultures that foster resilience and support people in their roles.

Examples of primary strategies include making sure that job roles include enough variation in their level of demand, so periods of intense involvement alternate with quieter times. High-risk staff groups may benefit from rotational work. Performance management systems should be designed to pick up early signs of stress and burnout, and managers should be trained to consider staff stress and the possibility of burnout in management supervision. Also helpful is a culture of regular, high quality supervision and a good upwards management structure (i.e. enabling staff to access and influence decisions at higher management levels in the organisation). Managers should also work actively with their teams to ensure a supportive culture where people take care of themselves – going home on time, taking lunch breaks, and supporting each other emotionally.

Secondary prevention involves setting up systems of early identification of problems, and initiatives such as flexible hours, and staff training. Examples include flexible working such as job sharing, training for staff in areas such as time management, stress management and assertiveness, as well as support to employees in managing their workloads through the effective use of technology.

At the third level of intervention, therapeutic care, employee assistance programmes and occupational health services provide intervention and rehabilitation for people who are suffering from stress and burnout.

REFLECTIVE ACTIVITY

What are the strategies that your organisation has employed to assist its workforce in managing stress? For example, are there policies on supervision, work-related stress, and occupational health? Also think about working practices such as the following:

- Clinical and management supervision

- Appraisals

- Organisational culture in areas such as participation in decision making and working hours

- Making information on stress and the available sources of support such as occupational health easily accessible to staff

- Skills training.

To help you think about how your organisation supports its staff, try to draw up a table of the primary, secondary and tertiary strategies for stress prevention and management that you can identify. Also consider the following questions:

1. What are your responsibilities as an employee? What is the role of your manager?

2. Looking at all three levels of intervention, how can reflective practice play a role in combating the impact of stress and burnout?

THE ROLE OF REFLECTIVE PRACTICE IN COMBATING STAFF STRESS

How would engaging in regular reflective practice support staff in frontline services to deal more effectively with issues of stress and burnout? As we have seen earlier, the experience of stress is dependent on individuals' appraisals of threat within the situations they encounter. Through developing a language that fosters an understanding of the psychological impact of the work in frontline settings, as we have done for much of this book, practitioners may find that they approach situations that they have found frustrating, puzzling or distressing in the past, with more understanding. This may mean that some situations you found stressful in the past may not be so stressful once you have a framework for understanding what is happening and the ability to reflect on how you are personally affected.

Regularly engaging with your own reactions to your work life allows you to become aware of growing feelings of unease or distress before you reach a crisis point. Reflecting with others allows you to mobilise support early on, before burnout becomes a risk. There may also be a benefit in writing down or drawing your feelings and experiences at work – much as the extended examples in this book have illustrated. This enables you to articulate and refine how you explain situations to yourself. Using the CLT framework we have used throughout this book is a further useful tool in making explicit your reflections on your own sources of stress at work.

There is also a benefit to teams in that practitioners can give each other peer support and provide one another with a way to achieve early warning of impending difficulties. When teams reflect together, this presents them with unique opportunities for developing solutions to sources of stress that lie in the way they structure their work flow. There may be opportunities to feed their solutions back into their organisations, thus improving practice on a larger scale. When all is not well, organisations that positively encourage reflective practice among their staff benefit from the early warning signals that reflective practitioners can generate, either through their personal supervision or through feedback built into the way reflective practice is embedded in the organisation.

Finally, reflective practices provide ways for frontline practitioners to make sense of what they experience and to vent their emotional reactions to the work. If reflection is practised regularly and in a team context, then staff stresses and anxieties can be contained and managed in a timely way. From an organisational perspective, this means that the service becomes a holding environment not only for service users, but also for practitioners.

FOR THE JOURNAL

In your journal, draw a map that shows how you feel about your job or study course right now. What are the positives and the stressors? Where does your support come from? What difference would regular time for team reflective practice make to your situation?

The example map below is for a student social worker on placement in a family support team.

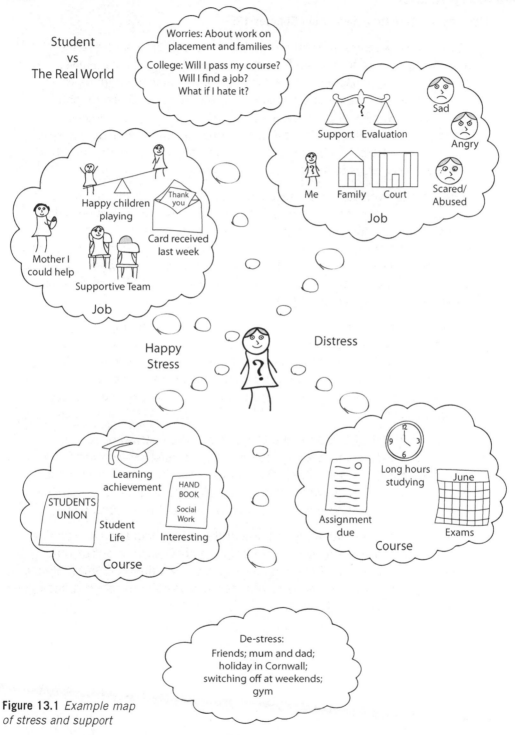

Figure 13.1 *Example map of stress and support*

CHAPTER SUMMARY

Five key points to take away from Chapter 13:

- Unhealthy work stress in frontline services occurs when practitioners' roles demand more from them than they perceive they are able to give. This definition emphasises the personal and interactional nature of stress: it is frontline practice contexts which make the demands on them, and practitioners who experience these as exceeding their capacity to cope, leading to them feeling under stress. Reflective practice can help you spot early signs of stress in yourself and enable you to come up with innovative and meaningful ways to manage your work stress.

- Humans have evolved a stress response that involves both the central nervous system and the endocrine system. The human stress response is designed to respond to environmental danger and prepare individuals for fight, flight or freeze reactions. These systems work well when activated in situations of acute, relatively short-lived threat, but, when chronically activated – as in situations of ongoing work stress – the stress response is likely to become unhelpful and may lead to long-term adverse health consequences.

- In extreme cases of stress, especially within the caring or helping professions, burnout can follow a period of chronic work stress. Burnout is generally characterised by the following three symptoms: extreme fatigue and depression (lack of motivation), a diminished sense of personal accomplishment (loss of confidence), and a sense of depersonalisation (feeling distant).

- Individuals with high need for approval and achievement, who are unassertive, and who need always to be on top of things or in control, are especially at risk for burnout, although anyone who is exposed to very high levels of demand in their work roles can develop the symptoms of burnout. Practitioners in frontline services frequently fall into these categories.

- When supporting individuals with burnout the focus should be on providing social support, addressing key psychiatric symptoms such as anxiety and depression, and helping them find new sources of vitality which may include returning to work in a phased way, with new responsibilities, or even finding a new career direction to develop.

FURTHER READING

The Health and Safety Executive (HSE) in the UK has produced a number of excellent online materials about stress and sickness absence in the workplace. The HSE website (www.hse.gov.uk) contains research reports and practical tools that organisations can use to support their policies around stress at work.

If you would like to find out more about burnout, and how to recognise and support individuals who have burnt out, there are a number of excellent books available by Christina Maslach and her co-workers who have made extensive studies of burnout in the caring professions. A good starting point would be Maslach's book *Burnout: The Cost of Caring*, referenced in this chapter.

EXTENDED EXAMPLE 4

REFLECTING ON STRESS, SUPERVISION AND TEAM SUPPORT

Suria is a Parenting Support Advisor (PSA), splitting her time between three primary schools, one of which has a nursery attached. She has been in her post for nine months and is the first practitioner in this role, so when she started it was not very clear what the role would entail. The learning curve for her and the schools was steep. She has monthly supervision with one of the County Specialist Advisory Teachers who has knowledge of behaviour management in the classroom, but no experience supporting vulnerable families in their own homes around parenting, a key part of Suria's work.

Lately, Suria has been feeling more and more isolated and has become increasingly aware that she is struggling to keep her head above water. Her last two supervision sessions had to be postponed due to her supervisor's workload, and when they did happen, they felt very rushed to her. When she started in the post, all of the PSAs in the county met every couple of months to share experiences and train together. Now that the training programme has been completed, the meetings have fizzled out. Since starting in her post Suria has kept a reflective journal, a practice she continued from her training course. The following is an extract from her journal and shows how she used some of the techniques discussed in the previous chapters to help her make sense of what is happening for her in the workplace:

EXTRACT FROM SURIA'S JOURNAL

My questions:

I feel so stressed and demotivated; why?

I feel isolated in my job.

It seems to me that the schools expect me to do miracles with all their problem parents. Don't they understand my role is to support basic parenting in the home, not fix hopeless situations?

What difference do I really make?

Why do other agencies withdraw as soon as they find out I am on board?

My drawing

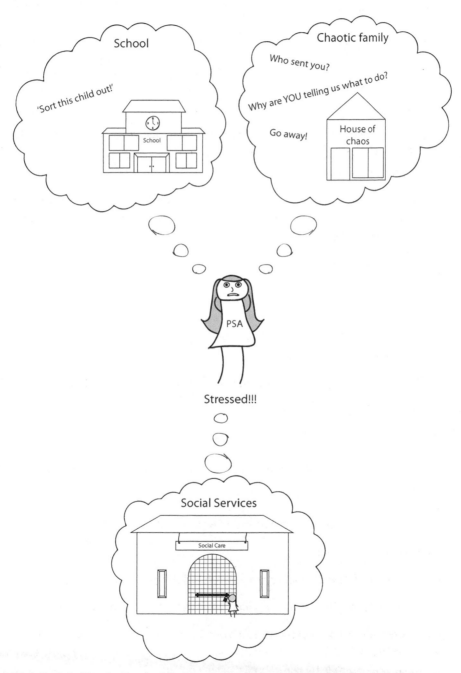

Figure E4.1 *Suria's illuminative incident analysis of her situation*

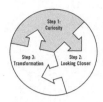

My CLT cycle

Curiosity and first attempts at looking closer:

Why am I feeling so tired and stressed? Some factors that affect my feelings are:

- The schools are demanding and expect me to perform miracles with problem children.

- A small number, but not all, of my families are hostile and uncooperative. I want to help them and they don't want help – this is very frustrating and feels like a slap in the face. It makes me feel useless.

- Social care seem very keen to get rid of cases and very eager to be able to say that the PSA has taken on a family. On the other hand, when I raise concerns about a family, nothing seems to happen.

- My manager has worked with behaviour in the classroom but not with families and it feels like supervision is very rushed and focuses on managerial elements, so I feel left out on a limb regarding difficult case work.

Some questions for personal reflection:

1. How do my feelings reflect what might be happening for the other agencies and people I work with?

2. Are there characteristics of my work and the way it is structured that make the problem worse?

3. How bad is it? Do I have stress symptoms or do I just feel overwhelmed?

4. What can I do about it?

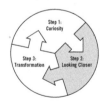

Looking closer:

1. How might my feelings be a mirror of what is happening around me?

I feel:

- Useless regarding my interventions

- Abandoned by my manager

- Under pressure to fix families and children from referring schools

- Powerless when faced with Social Services' reluctance to act on my concerns.

Perhaps these feelings reflect how useless, powerless and confused parents might feel when confronted with children who are disobedient and in trouble in school; they are made to feel ultimately responsible by the schools, given conflicting advice by different agencies and also they have no control over how teachers manage their children in the school setting. Perhaps their response to me makes me feel as powerless as they do, and it might prove to them that even the professionals can't fix it.

My manager is always busy and running around which means supervision is regularly postponed or rushed. I can never talk through any cases thoroughly with her, but perhaps that reflects also her feelings about the many aspects of her role – that she cannot attend to any of them with the level of intensity and time she would like to?

Schools put me under lots of pressure to fix families and this may reflect the pressures they face not to exclude pupils and get good academic results. They are hoping for miracles for the most disadvantaged or difficult to reach pupils.

Social workers in social services might feel huge pressure to close many cases; pressure to 'do something' or address risk; reluctant to take on new work as the work can be so demanding on top of huge existing workloads; aware of shortage of resources and help that is available to problem families.

So there are lots of bits of the system that are reflected in how I feel (I wonder if my colleagues feel the same, as I now work virtually alone).

2. My work role and its contribution to how I feel:

I work alone with my families; my referrals come from schools and I rarely get to meet with my colleagues in similar roles – so no one in the schools understands what situations I come across on a daily basis and no one else in my schools does a similar job. No wonder I started to feel really alone just after our regular PSA training days stopped!

Checklist for early signs of stress:

Table E4.1 *Suria's checklist for early signs of stress*

1	I find it hard to switch off from work while away from the office or when on holiday.	Yes
2	I have difficulty sleeping, due to worrying about work-related issues.	Yes
3	I have been more irritable than usual lately.	Yes
4	I dread going in to work on most days.	Yes
5	I am finding it very hard to make decisions.	No
6	I have been off sick more than usual in the last few months.	Yes
7	Nowadays I find myself working longer hours, but achieving less.	Yes
8	I have recently had incidents at work where I behaved out of character, for instance losing my temper with a client, subordinate or co-worker.	No
9	I have been drinking more than usual in the last few months.	No

| 10 | I have been experiencing more frequent physical symptoms than usual; for example, frequent headaches or abdominal pain. | No |

I have answered 'yes' to six out of ten early stress indicators which means I must be under some work stress – it certainly feels like it! Could I be starting to suffer from burnout?

Table E4.2 *Suria's checklist for early signs of burnout*

1	I almost always find myself with insufficient time to do things at work I actually enjoy.	No
2	I feel overwhelmed by the demands of my role.	Yes
3	I find it very difficult to get to sleep for worrying about work-related issues.	Yes
4	I panic or feel a strong sense of dread about going in to work.	Yes
5	I feel like I am starting to 'lose control' at work. For example, I am very indecisive and I do not see things in their proper perspective.	No
6	It feels like I am just going through the motions.	No
7	I am starting to feel my job is not worth while.	Sometimes I feel this way
8	I don't really make a difference to anyone in my job.	No
9	I have stopped caring; I've lost my passion and enthusiasm.	No
10	I am very prone to use procrastination as an avoidance strategy at work.	No

I've answered 'yes' to three and 'sometimes' to one out of the ten items, so I don't think I'm burnt out yet! But I think job stress is part of the problem for me at the moment and explains why I am so down and tired much of the time.

I also wonder about the PSA service as a team. Do we function well? I don't think so, but here is my systematic assessment on the team functioning checklist (see *Table 11.2*).

Table E4.3 *Suria's completed team functioning checklist*

Indicator	Rating (0–10)	What we can do to improve
1. A shared purpose or mission that is meaningful	4	We almost got there with our shared training days, but did not see things through when we stopped meeting together.

Indicator	Rating (0–10)	What we can do to improve
2. Clear, measurable goals	0	We have none. All PSAs are just appointed to their schools, we don't know what we are supposed to achieve as a group or how we contribute to larger goals in education.
3. A collaborative way of working together	7	We all help each other by sharing resources and talking informally when we have time. This is something we can build on.
4. Well-defined roles and responsibilities	6	We have job descriptions and made a start at educating the schools, but we don't have a single line of management and so everyone does things somewhat differently. This leaves us all confused about what is expected from us.
5. Everyone shares in the accountability	0	No. We don't experience any accountability except to our line managers and the schools who want us to see more and more families.
6. A willingness to learn/develop the team's functioning	9 (PSAs) Unsure (Employer)	We would like to develop as a team, but we are unsure if our employer wants us to or will support our efforts at this.
7. Participation in decision making and planning	0	We don't meet as a group and we don't have a say in anything about our jobs – or so it feels.
8. Passion and enthusiasm	8 but falling	My chats with others in similar roles tell me everyone is feeling a little overwhelmed right now and less enthusiastic than before.
9. Celebrating work well done together.	0	Never had a chance to do this yet.

I also feel my supervision is not working. We cover a lot of policy stuff, management matters and organisational information which all fall under the normative branch of supervision. But I need more input on how I am supposed to work with difficult families (formative supervision) and I want the time and space to talk through how I feel about my work and my own responses to the parents (restorative supervision).

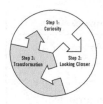

Transformation

Summary of what I have learned so far:

My feelings about my work reflect in some ways what is going on around me: social workers are overwhelmed and therefore delighted to pass on cases to me, but reluctant to take on my concerns, which makes me feel used and unimportant; families feel that my involvement is just one more professional telling them how to raise their children and my feelings of being useless at helping them may reflect their feelings of powerlessness at their children's behaviour and their powerlessness at the System which keeps telling them they've failed and chucks 'help' at them.

The demands on schools to get good league table results and include all children may be reflected in my feelings of being placed under a lot of unreasonable demands by schools.

My supervision feeling rushed, fragmented and unsupportive may be a reflection of my supervisor's fragmented and rushed job.

Into all of this feeds the fact that I am not part of a strong team where people can provide mutual support to each other.

Now I don't feel quite so hopeless. My reflections have lead to a number of things I can do to make the situation better. Here is my plan for the next three months:

1. Work with my fellow PSAs to become more of a team: ask all the managers if we can reinstate a meeting of PSAs every month to share best practice, feed back information, and talk about our roles.

2. Produce a leaflet with information on what we do for schools and social workers so they know what the referral criteria are and more or less what we are able to achieve.

3. Try to set up meetings with all my schools to explain the leaflet and talk through my role once again.

4. Ask my manager if we can spend some time talking about my supervision. My points will be about what I need in supervision, and I want to make sure she will meet my needs or allow me to be supervised by someone who can.

5. When I come across difficult situations such as very hostile families, try to find out what happened to them in the system that might explain their reactions and take that to supervision.

6. Be aware of my stress: I need to be better at taking lunch breaks and going home on time. Most admin tasks can wait until the morning!! I also need to look at my work–life balance and perhaps start a new hobby.

Discussion questions

1. What are your thoughts on the content and process of Suria's attempt at using structured reflective techniques to think through the difficulties she has been experiencing at work? (By content I mean the specific techniques she selected to help her make sense of her situation; process refers to the way she went about using and making sense of the techniques she chose to reach the resulting action plan.)

2. If you were to find yourself in a similar situation to Suria in terms of stress levels, what would your work situation look like? Do you have similar sources of stress in your work role?

3. Using your knowledge of reflective practice and the different reflective techniques you have encountered while working through this text, how would you go about making sense of the situation you described above?

4. A reflective process very rarely has a neat and tidy ending; neither does reflection always lead to finding satisfactory answers. In what ways is your reflective journey incomplete? What do you need to do to further the process of reflective practice for yourself?

FOR THE JOURNAL

Use your journal to engage in a reflective exercise with the aim of helping you make sense of your situation at work, in a similar way to what Suria did in this extended example. For instance, you might find that you are under similar levels of stress for different reasons, or perhaps even that you have cause to celebrate. In the latter case, what are the strengths in your team, organisation, the wider system and yourself that help you to thrive at work? One interesting question that is not included in the example given here, but that you can address using the material given in *Chapter 11*, is whether or not your team has a balance of team roles present, and what part you play in team functioning.

Following your reflection, what action steps have you come up with?

Once you have completed the task, reflect on the content and process that you used for the purpose.

Once you have completed each of the action steps, you can use the CLT cycle to assess whether you reached your goal and what further steps you can take.

REFLECTING IN PRACTICE: A FINAL WORD

You've come to the end of this book. During the course of the preceding chapters we've covered a range of material designed to help you on your journey towards developing effective reflective practice. Perhaps it is appropriate at this point to take a moment to think about what you've learned from working through the chapters of this book. Do you feel that you have developed your ability to take on a more reflective stance regarding your experiences both as a practitioner and as a person? Tony Ghaye writes about the five habits of reflection. A good litmus test of the extent to which this book has helped you would be to reflect critically on your personal development of these habits:

Habit 1: Reflecting on your values

Habit 2: Reflecting on your feelings

Habit 3: Reflecting on your thinking

Habit 4: Reflecting on your actions

Habit 5: Reflecting on context

(Ghaye, 2008, pp. 60–61).

How do you rate your development of these five habits? My sincere hope is that in the course of working through this book, you have embarked on a journey of consciously challenging yourself in all five of the areas mentioned above.

One of the key points made throughout this book has also been the idea that reflective processes are at once imperfect and incomplete. Even when we have completed a single CLT reflective cycle of curiously asking questions, looking closer at a situation and learning from reflection, and transformation of our thinking or practice, the experience we have reflected on is likely to become the subject of further reflective cycles in an iterative process that may need many cycles before it fully recedes into the background.

A key element of the transformation phase in almost all of the examples of CLT cycles offered in this book has been ways in which practitioners can bring their learning back to their teams. Collective learning and reflecting with others are important (and related) aspects of taking reflective practice to the next level. Once there is a critical mass of practitioners in any organisation or team who have individually mastered the five reflective habits mentioned above, it is highly likely that they would want to develop their teams or organisations into reflective teams and reflective organisations; in other words, develop a collective form of reflective practice that can serve as a powerful force for team learning and organisational transformation.

A detailed description of how you can achieve this is beyond the scope of this book, but here are some simple steps that might help to get you started in working towards building reflective teams and organisations. The first step is for you, as a practitioner, to maintain and develop your own reflective practice skills. Try to gain your line manager's endorsement and the authority to set aside time for reflection by mentioning this in your appraisal or personal development review if you have one. Keep writing your journal. Use some of the reflective techniques you learnt in this book to help your team solve problems in the workplace. Allow your reflective work to influence how you use case supervision, so that your supervisor can see the difference that a more reflective approach makes to your case work. Ask your team to join you for informal reflective sessions and tell other people in your organisation of the benefits. Through engendering a 'bottom up' process of transformation, involving a large number of people who own the process, you may be surprised at what you can achieve, especially when practitioners are able to articulate how reflective practice helped them become more proficient at their roles, and also served to improve practice in the service as a whole.

Finally, let me know about your progress and achievements. Please get in touch if you have any comments on the contents of this book. I am particularly interested to hear how your reflective practices have led to service improvements and positive change in your workplace. You are also welcome to feed back on the content of the chapters and exercises in this book and make suggestions for topics that you would like us to include in future editions. Contact me at natius@lanternpublishing.com.

REFERENCES

Ainsworth, M., Blehar, M., Waters, E. & Wall, S. (1978) *Patterns of Attachment: a Psychological Study of the Strange Situation.* Hillsdale, New Jersey: Lawrence Erlbaum.

Bamber, M. (2006) *CBT for Occupational Stress in Health Professionals.* Hove, East Sussex: Routledge.

Bandura, A. (1982) Self-efficacy mechanism in human agency. *American Psychologist,* **37(2):** 122–147.

Banks, S. (2006) *Ethics and Values in Social Work,* 3rd edition. Basingstoke, Hampshire: Palgrave Macmillan.

Beauchamp, T.L. & Childress, J.F. (2008) *Principles of biomedical ethics,* 6th edition. New York: Oxford University Press.

Belbin, R.M. (2010) *Team Roles at Work,* 2nd edition. London: Butterworth-Heinemann.

Berne, E. (1975) *What Do You Say After You Say Hello?* London: Corgi Books.

Bertalanffy, L. von (1950) An outline of general system theory. *British Journal for the Philosophy of Science,* **1(2):** 134–165.

Bhugra, D. & Jones, P. (2001) Migration and mental illness. *Advances in Psychiatric Treatment,* **7(3):** 216–223.

Bishop, G.D. (1994) *Health Psychology: Integrating Mind and Body.* Boston, USA: Allyn and Bacon.

de Board, R. (1978) *The psychoanalysis of organisations.* London: Routledge.

Booth, T. (2000) Parents with learning difficulties, child protection and the courts. *Representing Children,* **13(3):** 175–188.

Booth, T. & Booth, W. (1994) Parental adequacy, parenting failure and parents with learning difficulties. *Health and Social Care in the Community,* **2(3):** 161–172.

Boros, S. (2009) *Exploring Organisational Dynamics.* London: Sage.

Brown, E. (1998) The transmission of trauma through caretaking patterns of behaviour in Holocaust families: re-enactments in a facilitated long-term second-generation group. *Smith College Studies in Social Work,* **68(3):** 270–285.

Byng-Hall, J. (1995) *Rewriting Family Scripts: Improvisation and Systems Change.* London: Guilford Press.

Casement, P. (1985) *On Learning From the Patient.* London: Routledge.

Children Act (1989) London: Her Majesty's Stationery Office.

Cortazzi, D. & Roote, S. (1975) *Illuminative Incident Analysis*. London: McGraw Hill.

Cuthbert, S. & Quallington, J. (2008) *Values for Care Practice*. Exeter: Reflect Press.

Department of Health (2001) *Valuing People: A New Strategy for Learning Disability for the 21ˢᵗ Century*. London: The Stationery Office.

Department of Health (2008) *Code of Practice Mental Health Act (1983)*. Published pursuant to Section 118 of the Act. London: The Stationery Office.

Dewey, J. (1933) *How We Think*. Boston, USA: D.C. Heath.

DiClemente, C. & Prochaska, J. (1985) 'Processes and stages of change: coping and competence in smoking behavior change' in Shiffman, S. & Wills, T. (eds.), *Coping and Substance Abuse*, pp. 319–342. New York: Academic Press.

Eisenbruch, M. (1991) From post-traumatic stress disorder to cultural bereavement: diagnosis of Southeast Asian refugees. *Social Science and Medicine*, **33(6)**: 673–680.

Epstein, R.S. (1994) *Keeping Boundaries: Maintaining Safety and Integrity in the Psychotherapeutic Process*. Washington, DC: American Psychiatric Press.

European Federation of Psychologists' Associations (EFPA) (2005) *Meta-Code of Ethics*. Available at www.efpa.eu and from EFPA, Grasmarkt 105/18, B1000, Brussels, Belgium.

Freeman, E.M. & Couchonnal, G. (2006) Narrative and culturally based approaches in practice with families. *Families in Society*, **87(2):** 198–208.

Freud, S. (1958) 'The dynamics of transference' in *The Standard Edition of the Psychological Works of Sigmund Freud*, vol. 12, p 99. London: Hogarth Press.

Geddes, H. (2006) *Attachment in the Classroom*. London: Worth Publishing.

Ghaye, T. (2008) *Building the Reflective Healthcare Organisation*. Oxford: Blackwell.

Ghaye, T. & Lillyman, S. (2006) *Learning Journals and Critical Incidents*, 2ⁿᵈ edition. London: Quay Books.

Goodman, J. (1984) Reflection and teacher education: a case study and theoretical analysis. *Interchange*, **15:** 9–26.

Gordon Training (date unknown) *The competence matrix*. The organisation can be contacted at: www.gordontraining.com.

Health and Safety Executive (1999) *The Costs to Britain of Workplace Accidents & Work-related Ill Health in 1995/96*. HMSO: Norwich.

Health and Safety Executive (2004) *Managing Sickness Absence in the Public Sector*. London: Cabinet Office.

Health Professions Council (HPC) (2006) *Standards of Conduct, Performance and Ethics*. Available from www.hpc-uk.org and HPC, Park House, 184 Kennington Park Road, London, SE11 4BU.

Hess, R. & Handel, G. (1967) 'The family as a psychosocial organisation' in Handel, G. (ed.), *The Psychosocial Interior of the Family: A Sourcebook for the Study of Whole Families*, pp. 10–29. Chicago: Aldine Publishing Company.

Horwath, J. & Morrison, T. (1999) *Effective Staff Training in Social Care: From Theory to Practice.* Hove, East Sussex: Routledge.

Howe, D., Brandon, M., Hinings, D. & Schofield, G. (1999) *Attachment Theory, Child Maltreatment, and Family Support: A Practice and Assessment Model.* Basingstoke, Hampshire: Palgrave Macmillan.

Hughes, L. & Pengelly, P. (1997) *Staff Supervision in a Turbulent Environment: Managing Process and Task in Front-line Services.* London: Jessica Kingsley.

Hyman, B. & Pedrick, C. (2005) *The OCD Workbook,* 2nd edition. Oakland, California: New Harbinger Publications.

Inskipp, F. & Proctor, B. (1993) *The Art, Craft and Tasks of Counselling Supervision, Part 1. Making the Most of Supervision.* Twickenham: Cascade Publications.

Jasper, M. (2003) *Beginning Reflective Practice: Foundations in Nursing and Health Care.* Cheltenham: Nelson Thornes.

Kahn, W. (2005) *Holding Fast: The Struggle to Create Resilient Caregiving Organizations.* Hove, East Sussex: Brunner-Routledge.

Kast, V. (1995) *Folktales as therapy.* New York: Fromm Publishing.

Kellerman, N. (2001) Psychopathology in children of Holocaust survivors: a review of the research literature. *Israel Journal of Psychiatry & Related Sciences,* **38(1):** 36–46.

Kets de Vries, M. & Miller, D. (1984) *The Neurotic Organization.* San Francisco: Jossey Bass.

Kolb, D. (1984) *Experiential Learning: Experience as the Source of Learning and Development.* New Jersey: Prentice Hall.

Knott, C. & Scragg, T. (2007) *Reflective Practice in Social Work.* Exeter: Learning Matters.

Leher, P., Woolfolk, R. & Sime, W. (2007) *Principles and Practice of Stress Management,* 2nd edition. London: The Guilford Press.

Lewin, K. (1943) Defining the 'Field at a Given Time'. *Psychological Review,* **50:** 292–310.

Luft, J. & Ingham, H. (1955) The Johari window, a graphic model of interpersonal awareness. *Proceedings of the Western Training Laboratory in Group Development.* Los Angeles: UCLA.

Maslach, C. (1982) *Burnout: The Cost of Caring.* Englewood Cliffs, New Jersey: Prentice-Hall.

Mental Capacity Act (2005) London: The Stationery Office.

Miller, W. & Rollnick, S. (2002). *Motivational Interviewing,* 2nd edition. New York: The Guilford Press.

Milne, D. (2009) *Evidence-based Clinical Supervision.* Chichester: BPS Blackwell.

Nursing and Midwifery Council (NMC) (2010) *The Code: Standards of Conduct, Performance and Ethics for Nurses and Midwives.* Available from www.nmc-uk.org and the NMC, 61 Aldwych, London, WC2B 4AE.

Payne, V. (2001) *The Team-building Workshop: A Trainer's Guide.* New York: AMACOM Books.

Scaife, J. (2001) *Supervision in the Mental Health Professions: A Practitioner's Guide.* London: Routledge.

Schön, D. (1983) *The Reflective Practitioner: How Professionals Think in Action.* Aldershot, Hampshire: Ashgate.

Shapiro, J. (2002) Applications of narrative theory and therapy in the practice of family medicine. *Family Medicine,* **34(2):** 96–100.

Sween, E. (1998) The one-minute question: What is narrative therapy? Some working answers. *Gecko,* **(2):** 3–6.

Symington, J. & Symington, N. (1996) *The Clinical Thinking of Wilfred Bion.* London: Routledge.

Taylor, B. (2006) *Reflective Practice: A Guide for Nurses and Midwives,* 2nd edition. Maidenhead, Berkshire: Open University Press.

Teyber, E. (1992) *Interpersonal Process in Psychotherapy,* 2nd edition. Belmont, California: Brooks/Cole.

Todd, G. & Freshwater, D. (1999) Reflective practice and guided discovery: clinical supervision. *British Journal of Nursing,* **8(20):** 1383–1389.

Tripp, D. (1993) *Critical Incidents in Teaching: Developing Critical Judgement.* London: Routledge.

UNICEF (2009) *The State of the World's Children: Celebrating 20 Years of the Convention on the Rights of the Child.* New York: United Nations Children's Fund.

White, M. (2007) *Maps of Narrative Practice.* New York: Norton.

Winnicott, D.W. (1960) 'The theory of the parent infant relationship' in Winnicott, D.W. (1990) *The Maturational Process and the Facilitating Environment,* pp. 37–55. London: Karnac Books.

Winnicott, D.W. (1990) *The Maturational Process and the Facilitating Environment.* London: Karnac Books.

Winnicott, D.W. (2005) *Playing and Reality.* London: Routledge.

INDEX

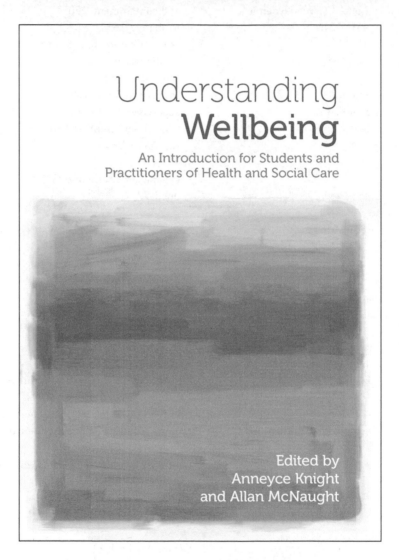

Understanding
Wellbeing

An Introduction for Students and
Practitioners of Health and Social Care

Edited by
Anneyce Knight
and Allan McNaught

Paperback – ISBN: 9781908625007

Titles of Related Interest

Communication and Interpersonal Skills

Elaine Donnelly; Lindsey Neville

Paperback – ISBN 9781906052065

Interpersonal Skills for the People Professions

Lindsey Neville

Paperback – ISBN 9781906052188

Understanding and Helping People in Crisis

Elaine Donnelly; Briony Williams; Tess Parkinson

Paperback – ISBN 9781906052218

Values for Care Practice

Sue Cuthbert; Jan Quallington

Paperback – ISBN 9781906052058